One-Stage Septic Revision Arthroplasty

Mustafa Citak • Mustafa Akkaya
Thorsten Gehrke
Editors

One-Stage Septic Revision Arthroplasty

Principles and Management

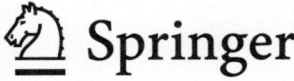

Editors
Mustafa Citak
Department of Orthopedic Surgery
Helios Endo-Klinik Hamburg
Hamburg, Germany

Mustafa Akkaya
Department of Orthopedic Surgery
Helios Endo-Klinik Hamburg
Hamburg, Germany

Thorsten Gehrke
Department of Orthopedic Surgery
Helios Endo-Klinik Hamburg
Hamburg, Germany

ISBN 978-3-031-59162-4   ISBN 978-3-031-59160-0   (eBook)
https://doi.org/10.1007/978-3-031-59160-0

© The Editor(s) (if applicable) and The Author(s), under exclusive license to Springer Nature Switzerland AG 2024

This work is subject to copyright. All rights are solely and exclusively licensed by the Publisher, whether the whole or part of the material is concerned, specifically the rights of translation, reprinting, reuse of illustrations, recitation, broadcasting, reproduction on microfilms or in any other physical way, and transmission or information storage and retrieval, electronic adaptation, computer software, or by similar or dissimilar methodology now known or hereafter developed.

The use of general descriptive names, registered names, trademarks, service marks, etc. in this publication does not imply, even in the absence of a specific statement, that such names are exempt from the relevant protective laws and regulations and therefore free for general use.

The publisher, the authors and the editors are safe to assume that the advice and information in this book are believed to be true and accurate at the date of publication. Neither the publisher nor the authors or the editors give a warranty, expressed or implied, with respect to the material contained herein or for any errors or omissions that may have been made. The publisher remains neutral with regard to jurisdictional claims in published maps and institutional affiliations.

This Springer imprint is published by the registered company Springer Nature Switzerland AG
The registered company address is: Gewerbestrasse 11, 6330 Cham, Switzerland

If disposing of this product, please recycle the paper.

Foreword 1

We Need Evidence: In All Its Forms

Evidence-based orthopedics informs decisions for the care of our patients. This approach refers to using the best clinical evidence to aid in patient care and, in turn, consider both physician expertise and the preferences of the patient. Evidence-based surgeons consider the hierarchy of evidence in all its forms, from systematic reviews to randomized trials. The point is that the totality of the information available should be considered, analyzed, and disseminated.

The more serious, and common, the health care issue the greater the care we must take to ensure a transparent, data-supported argument to support our recommendations. Periprosthetic joint infection (PJI) is an uncommon but devastating complication of patients undergoing total joint arthroplasty. Unquestionably, efforts to identify factors associated with the incidence, diagnosis, and treatment of PJI are critical. Drs. Citak, Akkaya, and Gehrke with a global community of experts present evidence and approaches to the management of PJI. Together, they have carefully curated the data and used their expertise to distill decades of information into practical recommendations for patient care.

This textbook serves as an important contribution to the field—and the ongoing discussion in the management of PJI. The hallmark of evidence-based orthopedics, after all, is to expose ourselves to all the evidence—and consider all approaches in optimal surgical care of patients.

Canada Research Chair in Surgical Innovation,   Mohit Bhandari
Department of Surgery, McMaster University,
Hamilton, ON, Canada

Foreword 2

One-Stage Exchange Arthroplasties: Principles and Management

Throughout my career, I have always had an interest in the diagnosis and treatment of Prosthetic Joint Infection (PJI). However, my passion for PJI hit close to home when I personally underwent a two-stage procedure for an infected knee. Going through this I experienced firsthand the problems of a two-stage solution to PJI, especially the psychological challenges for the patient struggling to recover from the first stage and having to look forward to another major procedure.

In addition to the morbidity of this approach, the economic ramifications of a two-stage approach warrant a reevaluation of the standard of care in the United States. To this end, 5 years ago we initiated a randomized trial of over 300 patients to determine if the results of a one-stage approach would be similar to the traditional two-stage approach.

We recently presented data at the 2024 American Academy of Orthopedic Surgeons meeting. Our 1-year comparative data between a one- and two-stage approach showed that the success of one-stage was 98% compared to 92% of those patients treated with a two-stage approach. While the one-stage data is encouraging, we cautioned our audience to not change their present practice patterns until we have 2-year data.

If in fact the one-stage results remain similar to two-stage treatment, a book of this nature will be a valuable addition and a real resource for surgeons contemplating moving to one-stage PJI treatment.

Atrium Musculoskeletal Institute, OrthoCarolina Thomas K. Fehring
Hip and Knee Center, OrthoCarolina Foundation,
Charlotte, NC, USA

Foreword 3

We have come a long way and yet not far at all. Over 20 years ago I became interested in periprosthetic joint infection. I started clinical and basic science research to address some of the issues that we were facing. When I reflect on the issues then and now, depressingly I come to realize that we have made little progress over the last two decades. Our patients still suffer a miserable life when handed the diagnosis of periprosthetic joint infection. They have to face surgical interventions, usually multiple of those, undergo long periods of antimicrobial treatment with their adverse consequences, and still face the risk of failure. Perhaps the only great progress that we have made, thanks mostly to the work of our European colleagues, in particular Dr. Thorsten Gehrke, is the shift towards one-stage exchange arthroplasty.

I recall a meeting that I attended over a decade ago when two renowned surgeons declared that one-stage exchange will NEVER be accepted in North America. Thankfully, they were both wrong. With the emergence of evidence, there has been a great shift towards one-stage exchange arthroplasty in the US and globally. I have personally been doing one-stage exchange over the last 5–6 years. We have come to realize that the outcome of one-stage exchange may not be much, if at all, inferior to two-stage exchange. Considering the advantage of a single operation and elimination of the interim stage, which is extremely disabling for our patients, it should not come to anyone as a surprise why one-stage exchange is gaining so much traction in the US. Europeans were way ahead of us!

The current book comes at a great juncture. Some of the issues related to one-stage exchange needs to be addressed and we need great authorities to address them for us. The editors of this book, namely Drs. Citak, Akkaya, and Gehrke, have the appropriate experience, knowledge, and authority to do just that. The 12 chapters that have been assembled provide guidance about causes of PJI, diagnosis of PJI (which I was fortunate to write), and surgical treatment of PJI. The chapters are concise, relevant, and provide state-of-the-art information.

Congratulations to my great friends who have edited a timely and worthy book. We should all read this book from cover to cover. Let us hope we will start to make some strides in the years to come and minimize the morbidity and mortality for our patients with PJI.

International Joint Center, Acibadem University Javad Parvizi
Istanbul, Turkey

Contents

The Philosophy of One-Stage Septic Exchange 1
Seper Ekhtiari, Mustafa Akkaya, Thorsten Gehrke, and Mustafa Citak

Risk Factors for the Development of a Periprosthetic Joint Infection 9
Mustafa Akkaya, Marjan Wouthuyzen-Bakker, and Mustafa Citak

Diagnosis of Periprosthetic Joint Infection 23
Saad Tarabichi and Javad Parvizi

Multidisciplinary Team Management of Periprosthetic Knee Infections 33
Dia Eldean Giebaly, Andreas Fontalis, and Fares S. Haddad

Surgical Technique, Bone Loss, and Muscle Insufficiency 49
Bernd Fink

HIP; Surgical Technique: Bone Loss and Muscle Insufficiency 71
Akos Zahar, Nandor J. Nemes, and Christian Lausmann

Shoulder: Surgical Technique, Complications, and Results 83
Philip Linke and Jörg Neumann

Fungal Periprosthetic Joint Infection 99
Mustafa Akkaya, Serhat Akcaalan, and Mustafa Citak

Management of Reinfection After One-Stage Exchange Arthroplasty 105
Gerard A. Sheridan, Michael E. Neufeld, Andrea Volpin,
and Bassam A. Masri

Knee Arthrodesis: Salvage Procedure After Failed Total Knee Arthroplasty 119
Dhanasekara Raja Palanisami, Raja Bhaskara Rajasekaran,
Soundarrajan Dhanasekaran, Rithika Singh, Duncan Whitwell,
and Shanmuganathan Rajasekaran

Antimicrobial Therapy in One-Stage Revision Surgery 129
Anna Both, Flaminia Olearo, and Holger Rohde

Rehabilitation After One-Stage Septic Exchange 145
Johannes Reich

Contributors

Serhat Akcaalan Department of Orthopedic Surgery, Helios Endo-Klinik Hamburg, Hamburg, Germany

Mustafa Akkaya Department of Orthopedic Surgery, Helios Endo-Klinik Hamburg, Hamburg, Germany

Anna Both Institute for Medical Microbiology, Virology and Hygiene, University Medical Center Hamburg-Eppendorf, Hamburg, Germany

Mustafa Citak Department of Orthopedic Surgery, Helios Endo-Klinik Hamburg, Hamburg, Germany

Soundarrajan Dhanasekaran Department of Orthopaedics, Ganga Medical Centre & Hospitals Pvt. Ltd, Coimbatore, India

Seper Ekhtiari Department of Orthopedic Surgery, Helios Endo-Klinik Hamburg, Hamburg, Germany

Bernd Fink Department of Joint Replacement and Revision Arthroplasty, Orthopaedic Clinic Markgröningen, Markgröningen, Germany

Andreas Fontalis University College London Hospitals (UCLH), London, UK

Thorsten Gehrke Department of Orthopedic Surgery, Helios Endo-Klinik Hamburg, Hamburg, Germany

Dia Eldean Giebaly University College London Hospitals (UCLH), London, UK

Fares S. Haddad University College London Hospitals (UCLH), London, UK

Christian Lausmann Department of Orthopedic Surgery, Helios Endo-Klinik Hamburg, Hamburg, Germany

Philip Linke Department of Orthopedic Surgery, Helios Endo-Klinik Hamburg, Hamburg, Germany

Bassam A. Masri Department of Orthopaedics, University of British Columbia, Vancouver, BC, Canada

Nandor J. Nemes, MD St. George University Teaching Hospital, Szekesfehervar, Hungary

Michael E. Neufeld Department of Orthopaedics, University of British Columbia, Vancouver, BC, Canada

Jörg Neumann Department of Orthopedic Surgery, Helios Endo-Klinik Hamburg, Hamburg, Germany

Flaminia Olearo Institute for Medical Microbiology, Virology and Hygiene, University Medical Center Hamburg-Eppendorf, Hamburg, Germany

Dhanasekara Raja Palanisami Department of Orthopaedics, Ganga Medical Centre & Hospitals Pvt. Ltd, Coimbatore, India

Javad Parvizi International Joint Center, Acibadem University Hospital, Istanbul, Turkey

Raja Bhaskara Rajasekaran Department of Orthopaedics, Ganga Medical Centre & Hospitals Pvt. Ltd, Coimbatore, India

Shanmuganathan Rajasekaran Department of Orthopaedics, Ganga Medical Centre & Hospitals Pvt. Ltd, Coimbatore, India

Johannes Reich ENDO Rehabilitation Center GmbH, Hamburg, Germany

Holger Rohde Institute for Medical Microbiology, Virology and Hygiene, University Medical Center Hamburg-Eppendorf, Hamburg, Germany

Gerard A. Sheridan Department of Orthopaedics, University of British Columbia, Vancouver, BC, Canada

Rithika Singh Department of Orthopaedics, Ganga Medical Centre & Hospitals Pvt. Ltd, Coimbatore, India

Saad Tarabichi Rothman Orthopaedic Institute, Philadelphia, PA, USA

Department of Orthopaedic Surgery, Mayo Clinic, Scottsdale, AZ, USA

Andrea Volpin NHS Grampian, Aberdeen, UK

Duncan Whitwell Nuffield Orthopaedic Centre Headington, Oxford, UK

Marjan Wouthuyzen-Bakker Department of Medical Microbiology and Infection Prevention, University Medical Center Groningen, University of Groningen, Groningen, The Netherlands

Akos Zahar St. George University Teaching Hospital, Szekesfehervar, Hungary

The Philosophy of One-Stage Septic Exchange

Seper Ekhtiari, Mustafa Akkaya, Thorsten Gehrke, and Mustafa Citak

Total joint arthroplasty (TJA) is one of the most successful medical interventions performed today. Total hip arthroplasty (THA) was named the operation of the century by the Lancet [1], and both THA and total knee arthroplasty (TKA) have patient satisfaction rates of over 85% [2]. As well, both THA and TKA have been found to be highly cost-effective based on high-quality studies [3]. Nonetheless, these major surgeries carry risks of major complications, with periprosthetic joint infection (PJIs) being among the most common causes of revision surgery [4, 5]. While the absolute rates of PJI are low (0.5–2%) [6], the overall large volume of TJAs worldwide [7] mean PJI represents an important and challenging issue. Periprosthetic joint infections represent a devastating complication, with important implications for patients and a major burden on healthcare systems [8]. As such, the diagnosis and treatment of PJIs continues to be studied and discussed in the literature.

There are multiple described strategies to treat PJIs, and choice of strategy depends on surgeon and institutional protocols, patient characteristics and preferences, chronicity and severity of infection, and a range of other factors. With the exception of a small number of patients who are too unwell to undergo any surgery, the treatment for PJI almost always includes surgical intervention. The least invasive surgical method for treating PJI is Debridement, Antibiotics, and Implant Retention (DAIR), which involves thorough irrigation and debridement, usually with exchange of modular implants but retention of well-fixed implants [9]. There is debate around the role DAIR plays in the management of PJI; typically, this

S. Ekhtiari · M. Akkaya · T. Gehrke · M. Citak (✉)
Department of Orthopedic Surgery, Helios Endo-Klinik Hamburg, Hamburg, Germany
e-mail: seper.ekhtiari@medportal.ca; mustafa@drakkaya.com;
Thorsten.Gehrke@helios-gesundheit.de; mustafa.citak@helios-gesundheit.de

© The Author(s), under exclusive license to Springer Nature Switzerland AG 2024
M. Citak et al. (eds.), *One-Stage Septic Revision Arthroplasty*,
https://doi.org/10.1007/978-3-031-59160-0_1

strategy is reserved for acute infections. Outcomes are variable, and reported success rates vary widely, ranging from 11% to 100% [10, 11], though most studies report 50–65% infection control rates [12].

The two gold standard strategies for the treatment of PJI are one-stage exchange arthroplasty and two-stage exchange arthroplasty. The technique for two-stage revision was first described in 1983 by pioneering British orthopedic surgeon John Insall [13]. This strategy includes, at minimum, two-staged procedures. In the first stage, the prior implants are removed, a thorough irrigation and debridement is performed, and a temporary 'spacer' which incorporates antibiotic cement is implanted. The patient is then placed on intravenous antibiotics, typically for 6–8 weeks. This requires an extended initial hospital admission, the placement of a central venous catheter, and, depending on the antibiotics used, regular bloodwork. Following this period, some surgeons institute an "antibiotic holiday," followed by bloodwork and possibly a joint aspiration, before proceeding with the second stage. In the second stage, the spacer is removed, and definitive implants are placed [14]. Thus, the full two-stage process can involve two operations, a total of 2–3 months, prolonged parenteral antibiotics, and frequent visits to clinical environments. Infection eradication rates are variably reported, but typically range between 70% and 85% [15, 16].

The one-stage exchange arthroplasty was first introduced in the 1970s by Professor Hans-Wilhelm Buchholz at the ENDO-Klinik in Hamburg, Germany [17]. In a 10-year series of 583 patients, Buchholz et al. reported a 77% success rate after a first attempt one-stage exchange arthroplasty [18]. The one-stage protocol continues to be a mainstay at the ENDO-Klinik, accounting for over 85% of all PJI revisions to this date [17]. Interest in the one-stage exchange arthroplasty has increased in recent years [19], and recent high-quality evidence has not shown a clear difference in infection eradication rates between one-stage and two-stage exchange arthroplasty [20, 21].

Certain requirements must be in place before deciding to pursue one-stage exchange arthroplasty. At minimum, the causative organism must be known through culture from aspirate or open biopsy [17]. As well, the organism must be amenable to treatment with available local and systemic antibiotic therapy. Furthermore, the host must be able to tolerate this lengthy and complex surgery, and this includes the soft tissue envelope around the joint, which must be in reasonable condition. Indications and contra-indications are discussed in further detail later in this book.

The philosophy behind the one-stage exchange arthroplasty is multifaceted and starts with an understanding that the one-stage exchange arthroplasty is not simply a surgical technique, but rather a comprehensive, multidisciplinary, perioperative protocol, which starts with the first suspicion of infection, and extends well beyond the operating room into the post-operative follow-up period. This book will outline in detail each step of the process, starting with appropriate diagnosis, multidisciplinary involvement, detailed surgical technique, post-operative antibiotic and rehabilitation protocols, and salvage options. Overall, however, the philosophy behind the one-stage exchange arthroplasty can be thought of in terms of two broad categories: (1) the dangers of missed infection and (2) the potential benefits to be gained from a one-stage operation compared to two-stage exchange arthroplasty.

The Dangers of Missed Infection

Long before any consensus meetings were held to discuss the issue of PJIs, unrecognized infection was a topic of concern and discussion among arthroplasty surgeons in the 1970s and 1980s. Hunter et al., in a careful evaluation of a series of presumed aseptic revision THAs, reported that 32% of cases in fact turned out to be infected [22]. In their clinical series, Buchholz et al. refer to this paper with an ominous warning: *"The dangers of unrecognised infection at revision arthroplasty should not be underestimated"* [18]. While certainly applicable to presumed aseptic revision TJA, this ethos also forms the basis of the philosophy behind one-stage exchange arthroplasty.

At its core, one-stage exchange arthroplasty operates on the principle that, if every effort is made to identify, remove, and treat the causative organism of the infection, then a one-stage exchange arthroplasty should be successful in most cases. This principle must be applied at each stage of the process. At the diagnosis stage, this means not missing a diagnosis of infection, including latent, subclinical, and low-grade infections which may not present classically. This demands a rigorous diagnostic workup, including prolonged culture times to avoid missed diagnosis of slow-growing organisms [23], and a high index of suspicion when faced with negative aspirate results despite a clinical picture consistent with PJI. The ENDO-Klinik protocol includes aspiration of *all* revision arthroplasties, even if they are presumed aseptic; as well, the protocol includes aspiration of all other prosthetic joints a patient has if a diagnosis of PJI is established—unrecognized synchronous infections can act as an occult source of infection, seeding recurrent infections in the revised joint [24]. The diagnostic principles and process are discussed in detail in chapter "Diagnosis of Periprosthetic Joint Infection".

The entire process also demands a close working relationship with a range of other healthcare providers, including microbiologists, operating room staff, nursing, physiotherapy, and others. While "multidisciplinary approach" is a vogue term that has garnered much attention and discussion in recent years, the meaning of the term has long been a part of the one-stage exchange arthroplasty philosophy—Prof. Buchholz worked closely with the microbiologist Prof. Lodenkämper, who was also a co-author on their 10-year clinical series discussed earlier [18]. The importance of the multidisciplinary nature of this technique is discussed in chapter "Multidisciplinary Team Management of Periprosthetic Knee Infections".

The philosophy of leaving no infection behind is perhaps most obviously and concretely applied in the operating room, the details of which are discussed in detail in chapters "Surgical Technique, Bone Loss, and Muscle Insufficiency" and "HIP; Surgical Technique: Bone Loss and Muscle Insufficiency". As per the original

Buchholz technique, previous scars and sinuses are excised, and the key concept here is radical debridement—*"the aim is to excise radically all infected or devascularized scar tissue and necrotic bone"* [18]. As Prof. Buchholz himself pointed out, no two cases are identical [18], and experience in managing PJI is critical in judging the amount of excision required—regardless, one must remember the goal here is to leave no infected tissue behind, in other words, 'leave no stone unturned'. The old surgical adage of 'if in doubt, cut it out' may be applied cautiously and expertly here.

Despite all best efforts and rigorously applied protocols, a perfect infection eradication rate is not realistic—at least not at the present time. Thus, understanding how to diagnose and manage recurrent infection is a critical aspect of the process. This also speaks to the importance of patient expectations—patients must be counseled thoroughly and accurately on the possibility of recurrent infection, and what that may mean for them. This is true regardless of if the patient is treated with DAIR, one-stage, or two-stage revision. These issues are discussed in chapters "Management of Reinfection After One-Stage Exchange Arthroplasty" and "Knee Arthrodesis: Salvage Procedure After Failed Total Knee Arthroplasty".

The Benefits of One-Stage Exchange Arthroplasty

When it was first introduced by Prof. Buchholz, one-stage exchange arthroplasty was one way in which to attempt to deal with a difficult problem, and the knowledge was shared with the surgical community in hopes of helping other surgeons facing a similar situation. This was nearly a decade before Drs. Gordon Guyatt and David Sackett from McMaster University coined the term 'Evidence-Based Medicine' [25], and before the many changes in the technology, implants, and perioperative protocols of TJA which have taken place in the last 30+ years. While the underlying philosophy remains largely the same, the lens with which we evaluate one-stage exchange arthroplasty, and the volume of data and clinical cases available for us to do so, has expanded considerably.

Though the concept has been for a long time, it is no secret that modern medicine has only very recently begun to seriously incorporate a patient-centered approach to healthcare. Within arthroplasty, a patient-centered approach is almost inherent, given that the very disease being treated is most commonly being treated due to its impact on the patient's quality of life, and thus, patient preferences are almost inevitably included in the decision making. Prof. Buchholz, in his clinical series, outlines the importance of patient function—*"Exchange arthroplasty is not justified in terms of eradication of infection alone: the functional result and its duration are important"* [18]. When comparing two interventions in today's paradigm, it is essential to consider the differential impact of each intervention on patient function and quality of life.

Early evidence has demonstrated similar performance of one-stage exchange arthroplasty compared to two-stage in terms of patient-reported outcomes [26]. A recent RCT comparing one- to two-stage exchange arthroplasty reported significantly better function in the one-stage group in the first 3 months post-operatively, with no difference thereafter [21]. Future studies are needed to further investigate this topic, and patient preferences must be explicitly examined—if functional outcomes are similar, and potentially better with one-stage exchange in the short-term, which of the protocols described above would patients likely prefer? This question can only be definitively answered empirically with rigorous methodology.

Health economics is another field which has grown massively since the introduction of the one-stage protocol and must be considered when comparing interventions—in fact, many governmental research funding organizations require this to be a planned component of any new randomized controlled trial (RCT) proposal. The economic burden of PJI in the USA is projected to reach nearly $2 Billion USD by 2030 [27]; thus, the evaluation of any PJI intervention must consider its economic impacts. Limited evidence exists on the economics of one-stage versus two-stage exchange arthroplasty, though recent studies have begun to evaluate the topic. A recent RCT comparing one-stage to two-stage exchange arthroplasty demonstrated that a one-stage strategy was cost-effective over the two-stage strategy, at an incremental net monetary benefit of £11,167 [21]. As well, a retrospective cohort demonstrated no significant difference in quality-adjusted life years (QALYs) between the two strategies [26]. Another potential benefit of the one-stage strategy has recently come to light—the COVID-19 pandemic has demonstrated the tenuous state of many healthcare systems across the world, as well as the potential benefits of limiting contact with healthcare environments as much as possible. A well-established one-stage protocol may be more sustainable in the face of future similar events and may be a safer strategy overall for vulnerable patients [28].

Conclusion

"The dire results of infection involving an implant fixed by means of acrylic cement were appreciated as early as 1965" [18]. These words ring as true today as they did when Prof. Buchholz used them to start his landmark study, published in 1981. There remains no single "silver bullet" solution to PJI—even the diagnosis of PJI remains elusive at times. Nonetheless, great strides have been made in orthopedics, infectious disease, and evidence-based medicine since then, and the ability to collaborate on a global level represents an opportunity to continue to advance the science of PJI management while adhering to the sound principles and philosophy of infection management.

References

1. Learmonth ID, Young C, Rorabeck C. The operation of the century: total hip replacement. Lancet. 2007;370:1508.
2. Hamilton DF, Lane JV, Gaston P, Patton JT, MacDonald D, Simspon AHRW, et al. What determines patient satisfaction with surgery? A prospective cohort study of 4709 patients following total joint replacement. BMJ Open. 2013;3:e002525.

3. Daigle ME, Weinstein AM, Katz JN, Losina E. The cost-effectiveness of total joint arthroplasty: a systematic review of published literature. Best Pract Res Clin Rheumatol. 2012;26(5):649–58. http://linkinghub.elsevier.com/retrieve/pii/S1521694212000964.
4. Bozic KJ, Kurtz SM, Lau E, Ong K, Vail DTP, Berry DJ. The epidemiology of revision total hip arthroplasty in the United States. J Bone Joint Surg Am. 2009;91:128–33.
5. Ulrich SD, Seyler TM, Bennett D, Delanois RE, Saleh KJ, Thongtrangan I, et al. Total hip arthroplasties: what are the reasons for revision? Int Orthop. 2008;32:597.
6. Ahmed SS, Haddad FS. Prosthetic joint infection. Bone Joint Res. 2019;8(11):570–2.
7. Sloan M, Premkumar A, Sheth NP. Projected volume of primary total joint arthroplasty in the U.S., 2014 to 2030. J Bone Joint Surg Am. 2018;100:1455.
8. Kurtz SM, Lau E, Watson H, Schmier JK, Parvizi J. Economic burden of periprosthetic joint infection in the United States. J Arthroplasty. 2012;27(8 Suppl):61.
9. Qasim SN, Swann A, Ashford R. The DAIR (debridement, antibiotics and implant retention) procedure for infected total knee replacement—a literature review. SICOT J. 2017;3:2.
10. Tsang STJ, Ting J, Simpson AHRW, Gaston P. Outcomes following debridement, antibiotics and implant retention in the management of periprosthetic infections of the hip: a review of cohort studies. Bone Joint J. 2017;99B:1458.
11. Kunutsor SK, Beswick AD, Whitehouse MR, Wylde V, Blom AW. Debridement, antibiotics and implant retention for periprosthetic joint infections: a systematic review and meta-analysis of treatment outcomes. J Infect. 2018;77:479.
12. Nurmohamed FRHA, van Dijk B, Veltman ES, Hoekstra M, Rentenaar RJ, Weinans HH, et al. One-year infection control rates of a DAIR (debridement, antibiotics and implant retention) procedure after primary and prosthetic-joint-infection-related revision arthroplasty—a retrospective cohort study. J Bone Jt Infect. 2021;6(4):91.
13. Insall JN, Thompson FM, Brause BD. Two-stage reimplantation for the salvage of infected total knee arthroplasty. J Bone Joint Surg Am. 1983;65(8):1087.
14. Kuzyk PRT, Dhotar HS, Sternheim A, Gross AE, Safir O, Backstein D. Two-stage revision arthroplasty for management of chronic periprosthetic hip and knee infection: techniques, controversies, and outcomes. J Am Acad Orthop Surg. 2014;22(3):153.
15. Gomez MM, Tan TL, Manrique J, Deirmengian GK, Parvizi J. The fate of spacers in the treatment of periprosthetic joint infection. J Bone Joint Surg Am. 2015;97(18):1495–502.
16. Corona PS, Vicente M, Carrera L, Rodríguez-Pardo D, Corró S. Current actual success rate of the two-stage exchange arthroplasty strategy in chronic hip and knee periprosthetic joint infection. Bone Joint J. 2020;102-B(12):1682.
17. Gehrke T, Zahar A, Kendoff D. One-stage exchange: it all began here. Bone Joint J. 2013;95-B(11 Suppl A):77.
18. Buchholz HW, Elson RA, Engelbrecht E, Lodenkämper H, Röttger J, Siegel A. Management of deep infection of total hip replacement. J Bone Joint Surg Am. 1981;63(3):342.
19. Rowan FE, Donaldson MJ, Pietrzak JR, Haddad FS. The role of one-stage exchange for prosthetic joint infection. Curr Rev Musculoskelet Med. 2018;11:370.
20. Goud AL, Harlianto NI, Ezzafzafi S, Veltman ES, Bekkers JEJ, van der Wal BCH. Reinfection rates after one- and two-stage revision surgery for hip and knee arthroplasty: a systematic review and meta-analysis. Arch Orthop Trauma Surg. 2021;143:829.
21. Blom AW, Lenguerrand E, Strange S, Noble SM, Beswick AD, Burston A, et al. Clinical and cost effectiveness of single stage compared with two stage revision for hip prosthetic joint infection (INFORM): pragmatic, parallel group, open label, randomised controlled trial. BMJ. 2022;379:e071281.
22. Hunter GA, Welsh RP, Cameron HU, Bailey WH. The results of revision of total hip arthroplasty. J Bone Joint Surg Br. 1979;61(4):419.
23. Tarabichi S, Goh G, Zanna L, Qadiri Q, Baker C, Gehrke T, et al. Time to positivity of cultures obtained for periprosthetic joint infection. J Bone Joint Surg. 2022;105:107.
24. Thiesen DM, Mumin-Gündüz S, Gehrke T, Klaber I, Salber J, Suero E, et al. Synchronous periprosthetic joint infections: the need for all artificial joints to be aspirated routinely. J Bone Joint Surg Am. 2020;102(4):283.

25. Sackett DL, Rosenberg WMC, Gray JAM, Haynes RB, Richardson WS. Evidence based medicine: what it is and what it isn't. Clin Orthop Relat Res. 1996;455:3–5.
26. Budin M, Abuljadail S, Traverso G, Ekhtiari S, Gehrke T, Sommer R, et al. Comparison of patient-reported outcomes measures and quality-adjusted life years following one- and two-stage septic knee exchange. Antibiotics. 2022;11(11):1602.
27. Premkumar A, Kolin DA, Farley KX, Wilson JM, McLawhorn AS, Cross MB, et al. Projected economic burden of periprosthetic joint infection of the hip and knee in the United States. J Arthroplasty. 2021;36:1484.
28. Blandford A, Wesson J, Amalberti R, AlHazme R, Allwihan R. Opportunities and challenges for telehealth within, and beyond, a pandemic. Lancet Glob Health. 2020;8(11):e1364–5.

Risk Factors for the Development of a Periprosthetic Joint Infection

Mustafa Akkaya, Marjan Wouthuyzen-Bakker, and Mustafa Citak

Introduction

Total joint replacement (TJR) is performed to treat joint arthrosis in an increasing number of patients due to the advances in arthroplasty techniques. According to the American Joint Replacement Registry, a total of 2.4 million hip and knee arthroplasties were performed in 2021 and the number of hip and knee arthroplasties performed exhibited an 18.3% increase compared to the previous year [1]. Along with the said increase in the number of TJRs, a parallel increase was observed in the rate of periprosthetic joint infections (PJI), the most feared complication of joint replacement. Therefore, determining the risk factors for PJI would be effective in reducing the rate of this increase. In this context, the risk factors of PJI can be divided into two groups, wherein the first group consists of patient-related factors and the second group consists of surgery-related factors. The latter can also be divided into three subgroups, i.e., preoperative, intraoperative, and postoperative factors. This section will focus on patient—(Table 1) and surgery-related factors (Table 2) associated with PJI in detail.

Table 1 Patient-related factors associated with periprosthetic joint infection

Patient-related factors	
Non-modifiable factors	Modifiable factors
Age	Obesity
Gender	Smoking, alcohol, and intravenous drug use
Race	Active pyogenic infections
Socioeconomic status	Hyperglycemia and diabetes mellitus
Previous surgeries	Immunosuppression and autoimmune/rheumatic diseases
	Human immunodeficiency virus (HIV) infection

Table 2 Surgery-related factors associated with periprosthetic joint infection

Surgery-related factors		
Preoperative	Intraoperative	Postoperative
Skin shaving	The joint to be operated	Prolonged wound drainage
Antimicrobial prophylaxis	Revision surgeries	Problems related to the surgical wound
Skin antisepsis	Operative time	Allogeneic blood transfusion
Surgical scrubbing	Previous procedure in the operating room	Length of hospital stay
Surgical drapes, gloves, and gowns	Administration of anesthesia	
Operating room traffic		
Surgical instruments		

Patient-Related Factors

TJR has become applicable in various complex patient groups due to the advances in TJR techniques. However, patient characteristics directly affect the incidence of PJI, which remains to be the most important problem. In particular, patient comorbidities are known to alter the risk of PJI considerably. Therefore, a careful preoperative evaluation and optimization with a multidisciplinary approach are of critical importance in patients who are candidates for joint replacement. Patient-related factors can be grouped as modifiable and non-modifiable factors.

Non-modifiable Factors

These factors, which are evaluated preoperatively, can indicate that a patient is at increased risk for PJI. However, a benefit–risk assessment should be made before the decision to perform joint replacement, since these factors cannot be modified.

Age

The association between PJI and age is controversial. Studies in the literature have reported advanced age as a cause of PJI [2, 3]. In a study by Kurtz et al., it was demonstrated that PJI exhibited a bimodal distribution in patients aged 55–74 [4]. In addition, a study conducted in England showed that the patients aged 80 and over had increased risk of infection following total hip replacement (THR) [5]. However, a relationship has not been clearly demonstrated between PJI and age according to the arthroplasty registries [6, 7]. Bias and differences between studies and studied populations should be taken into account, since PJI is associated with comorbidities a factor that is more pronounced in the elderly population.

Gender

Many diseases of the musculoskeletal system differ between males and females due to the different effects of sex hormones and chromosomes on immune response [8]. Therefore, males and females respond differently to various pathogens, wherein the distribution of infection also exhibits a difference between genders. Numerous studies have shown that males have a higher risk of PJI compared to females [9–11]. On the other hand, considering both gender and obesity, the risk of PJI was found to be considerably higher in women. Factors relating to the association between PJI and gender were reported to be pH value in the skin, skin-subcutaneous fat layer thickness, body fat distribution, and metabolic rate. In addition, males are more likely to be *S. aureus* carriers [12].

Race

According to the literature, the incidence of early-onset PJI following TJR was shown to be higher in the nonwhite population [13–15]. However, this is also frequently associated with comorbidities, BMI and access to TJR. Considering all these, more extensive analyses are needed to obtain accurate data for a comparison between races.

Socioeconomic Status

The relationship between socioeconomic status and PJI is highly complicated. A lower socioeconomic status may have a potential impact on the risk of PJI, since it would negatively affect the general health status, self-care, and nutrition [9, 16–18]. However, evidence provided in the literature is not sufficient to clearly state that socioeconomic status is a factor in PJI.

Previous Surgeries

In the literature, it was demonstrated by several studies that previous surgeries in the knee and hip arthroplasty sites constitute a risk factor for PJI [19–21]. Therefore, a poorly planned skin incision and devitalized peri-incisional tissues may lead to increased surgical scar tissue complications. In a study by Werner et al., TKA performed within the first 6 months following knee arthroscopy was shown to be associated with an increased risk of PJI compared to the control group [22]. Similarly, a history of corticosteroid injections into the knee joint for less than 3 months was also associated with increased risk of PJI.

Modifiable Factors

Obesity
Obesity simultaneously triggers heart disease, hypertension, hypercholesterolemia, type 2 diabetes mellitus, and metabolic syndromes thereof, thereby leading to increased risk of comorbidities, postoperative recovery problems, and perioperative complications. This also points to an increased risk of PJI. Studies in the literature have shown that a BMI over 40 and 50 leads to 3.3- and 21-fold increased risk of PJI, respectively [23]. A BMI higher than 40 can be considered the cutoff value for arthroplasty [24]. In addition, studies have shown that a poorly vascularized thick subcutaneous adipose tissue leads to serious problems in recovery due to low oxygenation [25, 26]. Moreover, obesity is an important risk factor for nasal *S. aureus* carriage [27].

Smoking, Alcohol and Intravenous Drug Use
Smoking is a predisposing factor for infection due to its negative effects on the body's defense mechanism and tissue oxygenation. Studies have shown that smoking cessation 6–8 weeks prior to elective arthroplasty leads to a decreased risk of infection-related complications [28, 29]. However, the evidence has been mostly inconsistent regarding the association between smoking and risk of PJI following TJA. Strong evidence indicates that smoking cessation before surgery is linked to a 50% reduction in the incidence of postoperative infection [30].

Although moderate alcohol consumption was shown to have positive long-term effects on general health, it is known that excessive consumption of alcohol leads to an increase in various risks including the risk of surgical infection. This relationship was frequently attributed to an impairment in immunomodulatory mechanisms. However, more extensive studies are required regarding PJI.

Intravenous drug use is strongly associated with PJI development, with incidence rates over 25% in the literature [31]. Such patients are highly susceptible to candidemia and bacteremia, in particular to infections caused by *S. aureus*. Elective arthroplasty is contraindicated in these patients.

Active Pyogenic Infections
Active infections should be treated prior to elective arthroplasty. Today, elective arthroplasty is contraindicated in the presence of a known intraarticular infection, and implantation of a prosthetic should be postponed in case of doubt. Active skin infections lead to an increased risk of a potential PJI through adjacency. Infections disposes a higher risk for the development of bacteremia (tooth abscess, endovascular infections, pyelonephritis) are among the direct risk factors for PJI [32, 33].

Although odontogenic bacteremia is common among the elderly, it rarely causes hematogenous PJI. In the literature, there is no consensus on routine dental screening in patients undergoing arthroplasty. However, treatment should be initiated prior to elective arthroplasty in patients with focal dentogingival pain and infection.

Hyperglycemia and Diabetes Mellitus

Diabetes leads to a significantly increased risk of orthopedic infections. In addition, the literature shows that the risk of PJI is fourfold higher in patients with a glucose level higher than 7 mmol/L compared to those with a glucose level lower than 6 mmol/L [34, 35]. The latest consensus report on PJI also included a recommendation to include diabetes and glycemic control as part of routine screening [36].

Immunosuppression and Autoimmune/Rheumatic Diseases

Patients with autoimmune diseases usually have joint problems that require arthroplasty. Immunomodulators used by the patients and anatomical disorders lead to increased risk of infection [37, 38]. In such patients, a change in medication might be necessary after consulting the medical specialist that prescribed the medication in the preoperative period. In general, treatment with disease-modifying drugs is stopped before elective arthroplasty (the time of stopping treatment depends on the half-life) and restarted after a satisfactory progress is observed in wound healing.

Human Immunodeficiency Virus (HIV) Infection

According to the literature, HIV infection appears to be a very strong risk factor for PJI [39]. However, HIV-positive and HIV-negative patients were shown to have a similar PJI risk profile, when CD4 count was maintained over 200 with the current highly active antiretroviral therapies (HAART) in patients with HIV [40]. Therefore, HIV infection is not a significant risk factor for PJI in elective arthroplasty, provided that the patients are on HAART and the HIV is well controlled [41].

Surgery-Related Factors

Preoperative

The preoperative period is of utmost importance in terms of the surgery-related factors in PJI. Lister et al. explained the concept of antisepsis in surgery in 1867, after which Charnley et al. introduced the concept of clean air in 1960 [42]. Preoperative risk factors of infection include errors in skin preparation, preoperative antibiotic use, problems related to the operating room as well as problems related to the surgeon, surgical team, and equipment.

Skin Shaving

Preoperative shaving of the surgical site is common practice. However, bacterial growth can be observed on areas with microscopic abrasion, when shaving is performed a couple hours prior to surgery. In the literature, it was shown in a meta-analysis that using razors for preoperative shaving resulted in a significantly increased risk of infection compared to the use of clippers [43]. In addition, other studies have shown that shaving performed right before surgery led to a significantly lower rate of infection compared to shaving performed 24 or >24 h prior to surgery.

Antimicrobial Prophylaxis

Preoperative antibiotic prophylaxis leads to a lower risk of postoperative infection; therefore, it is used as part of standard practice in joint replacement surgery [44, 45]. There are certain recommendations about the selection of the antibiotic, prophylaxis duration, and timing of the first dose [46, 47]. In particular, beta-lactam antibiotics are usually preferred in TJA. It is known that administering the first dose as close as possible to the time of incision enhances the prophylactic effect. On the other hand, there is no consensus on the optimal duration of prophylaxis. According to the US advisory statement, antimicrobial prophylaxis should be administered 1 h prior to the incision and ceased within 24 h following the end of surgery [48]. On the contrary, European guidelines recommend administering a single dose within 30 min prior to the incision [49].

ICM recommends first- (e.g., cefazolin) or second-generation cephalosporins (e.g., cefuroxime) as the most suitable prophylactic antibiotics in patients undergoing primary TJA (strong consensus) [50]. In addition, American Academy of Orthopaedic Surgeons also included glycopeptide antibiotics (e.g., vancomycin) in the group of optimal prophylactic antibiotics in the clinical practice guidelines. On the other hand, various studies have shown that the use of antibiotics other than cefazolin in prophylaxis leads to an increased risk of PJI [51, 52]. Another important aspect is proper dosing of antibiotics. Administering low doses of antibiotics was associated with a high risk of PJI, wherein prophylactic antibiotic doses should always be based on weight [53]. The rate of cross-reactivity due to cephalosporin use is considerably low in patients who are allergic to penicillin [54, 55]. According to a recent study, cephalosporins can be safely used in 97% of the patients who are referred to an allergist due to an allergic reaction [51].

Skin Antisepsis

There are various preparations for surgical site preparation. The main goal is to reduce the number of microorganisms around the incision site. Iodophors, alcohol-containing products, and chlorhexidine gluconate (CHG) solution are among the most widely used agents. In a meta-analysis, there was no difference between clean surgeries in terms of the antiseptics used [56]. In addition, considering wound healing time, povidone-iodine (POI) was shown to be toxic to fibroblasts and keratinocytes, whereas chlorhexidine was shown to cause less irritation [57]. Moreover, the latest consensus report from the ICM emphasized that CHG bathing at home prior to orthopedic surgery was essential in reducing the risk of PJI [58].

Surgical Scrubbing

There is no clear view on surgical hand scrubbing in the literature. Studies have shown that there is no significant difference between alcohol-based solutions and POI or CHG in terms of infection rates [59]. ICM consensus report also did not provide a clear opinion and it was stated that antimicrobial soaps or alcohol-based hand sanitizers could be used [58]. While the adopted duration of scrubbing is generally 2–6 min, recommendations of the manufacturers should also be considered.

Surgical Drapes, Gloves, and Gowns

Surgical drapes are divided into two categories, i.e., cloth drapes and disposable plastic adhesive drapes. Plastic adhesive drapes were shown to reduce contamination [60]. However, a significant change in infection rates could not be demonstrated with the use of iodophor-impregnated drapes on the incision site [61].

Double gloving is common due to the risk of perforation, particularly in orthopedic surgery. Change of gloves in regular intervals would lead to a lower incidence of glove perforation and contamination.

Scientific studies have shown that disposable surgical drapes and gowns have the highest benefit-cost ratio [62]. However, it is recommended that surgeons avoid continuous contact with surgical gowns due to the large surface area of gowns and their contact with the environment.

Operating Room Setting

Although laminar air flow (LAF) was shown to reduce bacterial wound contamination, it failed to have a significant contribution to the reduction of infection rates. Therefore, a significant effect of LAF on PJI remains to be shown. In the ICM report, LAF was also supported by moderate level of evidence [63]. In addition, the use of ultraviolet (UV) light in the operating room is also effective against airborne bacteria. However, it is recommended to use UV light for the final cleaning when the operating room is empty, due to the risk it may pose to the OR personnel.

Operating Room Traffic

Healthcare personnel in the operating room is an important source of bacterial contamination. In addition, leaving the operating room doors open leads to an increased number of particles in the air. Therefore, operating rooms with open doors and a heavy healthcare personnel traffic are high-risk areas for PJI [64].

Surgical Instruments

Surgical instruments represent a potential source of infection. In particular, it was demonstrated that there is a positive correlation between the time surgical instruments are left exposed to the surrounding air and that the contamination rates were reduced when instruments were covered in case they were expected to be exposed for a long period of time [65]. Of note, splash basins, suckers, irrigation solutions, and light handles require special consideration, since these are the most commonly contaminated objects in the operative field.

Intraoperative

The Joint to Be Operated

Hip and knee replacements may not bear the same risk of PJI. Considering arthroplasty registries, the incidence rate of PJI is projected to exhibit a similar progressive increase within the same period of time in patients undergoing hip and knee replacements [66]. However, THA was associated with a consistently lower burden of PJI compared to TKA. In other studies, the incidence of infections was reported to be higher after tricompartmental compared to unicondylar knee replacement, wherein PJI incidence exhibited a threefold difference after 10 years of follow-up [67].

Revision Surgeries
Compared to primary joint replacement, revision surgeries were shown to be associated with a higher risk of infection in various studies [68]. In addition, it is known that the number of revision surgeries is directly proportional to the risk of PJI [69]. The relationship between PJI and revision surgeries can be confounded by factors such as prolonged operative time, comorbidities, higher incidence of postoperative wound complications and a higher need for blood transfusion. However, the relationship between revision arthroplasty and PJI still remained even when these factors were considered.

Operative Time
Operative time is defined as the time from skin incision to the end of skin closure. In the literature, this parameter was independently associated with PJI [70, 71]. Studies have described an arthroplasty procedure lasting 2–3 h as a prolonged procedure and found a significant relationship between operative time and PJI [72, 73]. Looking into primary and revision joint replacements separately, the incidence of PJI was shown to be significantly higher in procedures that took more than 2 h [5]. This increase is associated with an increased duration of contact with potential sources of contamination and the degree of tissue damage during surgery. This risk can be minimized by improving surgical techniques and assuring team unity as well as by increased surgical experience.

Previous Procedure in the Operating Room
There is no clear scientific evidence regarding the previous procedure performed in the OR. However, an infected case is generally operated after clean cases. The only study on this subject was performed with a limited case series of 39 patients [74]. Although there is no definitive evidence on cross-contamination, the risk still exists in theory and should not be ignored.

Administration of Anesthesia
Anesthesia directly affects tissue perfusion and immune response during surgery. Intraoperative hypothermia and hyperglycemia are known to impair tissue perfusion [75, 76], wherein decreased tissue perfusion and oxygenation are thought to increase the risk of PJI. In addition, it was demonstrated that hyperglycemia hinders neutrophil activation and disrupts bactericidal activity [77]. Considering the types of anesthesia, neuraxial anesthesia was shown to cause less peripheral vasoconstriction and it did not put additional pressure on immune response due to the lack of opioid use compared to general anesthesia. Therefore, neuraxial applications may pose a lower risk of PJI [78].

Postoperative

Prolonged Wound Drainage

Although there is no precise definition for prolonged wound drainage, wounds should be carefully monitored when drainage continues for more than 48–72 h [79]. Studies in the literature have shown that prolonged wound drainage, particularly for 5–7 days, is closely associated with PJI and causes up to 12-fold increased risk of infection [80]. Moreover, each day of prolonged drainage leads to a 40% and 30% increase in the probability of infection in hip and knee replacements, respectively [81]. Use of aspirin and warfarin for postoperative DVT prophylaxis has been linked to a shorter duration of drainage as compared to low molecular weight heparin [82].

Problems Related to the Surgical Wound

In general, a surgical intervention would not be necessary in case of complications related to surgical wounds such as wound dehiscence, wound edge necrosis, superficial infection, and delayed healing. However, it was demonstrated that these complications are linked to deep wound infection and lead to a fourfold increased risk of PJI within 5 years following knee arthroplasty [83, 84].

Allogeneic Blood Transfusion

Prevention of postoperative anemia constitutes great importance in many aspects and particularly for reducing the risk of PJI [85]. However, allogeneic blood transfusion, which is preferred when autologous blood products fail to suffice, may lead to increased risk of PJI as it alters the immune response [86]. ICM report also indicated that there was a strong relationship between allogeneic blood transfusion and increased risk of PJI [87].

Length of Hospital Stay

In the literature, there is no consensus or adequate level of evidence on the length of hospital stay. However, increased length of hospital stay is linked to an increased risk of PJI. In addition, a longer stay at the hospital may also point to a poor postoperative recovery, wherein noninfectious complications lead to an increased risk of joint contamination. In the context of PJI, the risk of contamination would be reduced when patients are discharged from the hospital environment. This idea is supported by the decreased rate of PJI among patients with a shorter length of stay at high-volume arthroplasty centers [88, 89]. However, length of hospital stay may vary depending on the sociocultural level of the patients, surgeon's preference and the hospital.

References

1. Siddiqi A, Levine BR, Springer BD. Highlights of the 2021 American Joint Replacement Registry Annual Report. Arthroplast Today. 2022;13:205–7.
2. Soohoo NF, et al. Factors that predict short-term complication rates after total hip arthroplasty. Clin Orthop Relat Res. 2010;468(9):2363–71.

3. SooHoo NF, et al. Factors predicting complication rates following total knee replacement. J Bone Joint Surg Am. 2006;88(3):480–5.
4. Kurtz SM, et al. Infection burden for hip and knee arthroplasty in the United States. J Arthroplast. 2008;23(7):984–91.
5. Ridgeway S, et al. Infection of the surgical site after arthroplasty of the hip. J Bone Joint Surg Br. 2005;87(6):844–50.
6. Matziolis G, Rohner E. [Total knee arthroplasty in 2014: results, expectations, and complications]. Orthopade. 2015;44(4):255–8, 560.
7. Havelin LI, et al. The Norwegian Arthroplasty Register: 11 years and 73,000 arthroplasties. Acta Orthop Scand. 2000;71(4):337–53.
8. Tosi LL, Boyan BD, Boskey AL. Does sex matter in musculoskeletal health? The influence of sex and gender on musculoskeletal health. J Bone Joint Surg Am. 2005;87(7):1631–47.
9. Ong KL, et al. Prosthetic joint infection risk after total hip arthroplasty in the Medicare population. J Arthroplast. 2009;24(6 Suppl):105–9.
10. Lenguerrand E, et al. Risk factors associated with revision for prosthetic joint infection after hip replacement: a prospective observational cohort study. Lancet Infect Dis. 2018;18(9):1004–14.
11. Willis-Owen CA, Konyves A, Martin DK. Factors affecting the incidence of infection in hip and knee replacement: an analysis of 5277 cases. J Bone Joint Surg Br. 2010;92(8):1128–33.
12. Sousa RJ, et al. Preoperative Staphylococcus aureus screening/decolonization protocol before total joint arthroplasty—results of a small prospective randomized trial. J Arthroplast. 2016;31(1):234–9.
13. Mahomed NN, et al. Rates and outcomes of primary and revision total hip replacement in the United States Medicare population. J Bone Joint Surg Am. 2003;85(1):27–32.
14. Ibrahim SA, et al. Racial/ethnic differences in surgical outcomes in veterans following knee or hip arthroplasty. Arthritis Rheum. 2005;52(10):3143–51.
15. Franklin PD, Suleiman L, Ibrahim SA. Racial/ethnic and sex differences in total knee arthroplasty outcomes. JAMA Netw Open. 2020;3(5):e205000.
16. DeKeyser GJ, et al. Socioeconomic status may not be a risk factor for periprosthetic joint infection. J Arthroplast. 2020;35(7):1900–5.
17. Maradit Kremers H, et al. Social and behavioral factors in total knee and hip arthroplasty. J Arthroplast. 2015;30(10):1852–4.
18. Bozic KJ, et al. Risk factors for early revision after primary total hip arthroplasty in Medicare patients. Clin Orthop Relat Res. 2014;472(2):449–54.
19. Peersman G, et al. Infection in total knee replacement: a retrospective review of 6489 total knee replacements. Clin Orthop Relat Res. 2001;392:15–23.
20. Klemt C, et al. Development of a preoperative risk calculator for reinfection following revision surgery for periprosthetic joint infection. J Arthroplast. 2021;36(2):693–9.
21. Li H, et al. The risk factors of polymicrobial periprosthetic joint infection: a single-center retrospective cohort study. BMC Musculoskelet Disord. 2021;22(1):780.
22. Werner BC, et al. Total knee arthroplasty within six months after knee arthroscopy is associated with increased postoperative complications. J Arthroplast. 2015;30(8):1313–6.
23. Malinzak RA, et al. Morbidly obese, diabetic, younger, and unilateral joint arthroplasty patients have elevated total joint arthroplasty infection rates. J Arthroplast. 2009;24(6 Suppl):84–8.
24. Foreman CW, et al. Total joint arthroplasty in the morbidly obese: how body mass index >/=40 influences patient retention, treatment decisions, and treatment outcomes. J Arthroplast. 2020;35(1):39–44.
25. Hopf HW, et al. Wound tissue oxygen tension predicts the risk of wound infection in surgical patients. Arch Surg. 1997;132(9):997–1004; discussion 1005.
26. Berrios-Torres SI, et al. Centers for disease control and prevention guideline for the prevention of surgical site infection, 2017. JAMA Surg. 2017;152(8):784–91.
27. Campbell KA, et al. Risk factors for developing Staphylococcus aureus nasal colonization in spine and arthroplasty surgery. Bull Hosp Jt Dis (2013). 2015;73(4):276–81.
28. Moller AM, et al. Effect of preoperative smoking intervention on postoperative complications: a randomised clinical trial. Lancet. 2002;359(9301):114–7.

29. Thomsen T, Villebro N, Moller AM. Interventions for preoperative smoking cessation. Cochrane Database Syst Rev. 2010;7:CD002294.
30. Sorensen LT. Wound healing and infection in surgery. The clinical impact of smoking and smoking cessation: a systematic review and meta-analysis Arch Surg. 2012;147(4):373–83.
31. Humphrey TJ, et al. Rates and outcomes of periprosthetic joint infection in persons who inject drugs. J Arthroplast. 2023;38(1):152–7.
32. Izakovicova P, Borens O, Trampuz A. Periprosthetic joint infection: current concepts and outlook. EFORT Open Rev. 2019;4(7):482–94.
33. Aalirezaie A, et al. Hip and knee section, prevention, risk mitigation: proceedings of international consensus on orthopedic infections. J Arthroplast. 2019;34(2S):S271–8.
34. Jamsen E, et al. Preoperative hyperglycemia predicts infected total knee replacement. Eur J Intern Med. 2010;21(3):196–201.
35. Godshaw BM, et al. Preoperative glycemic control predicts perioperative serum glucose levels in patients undergoing total joint arthroplasty. J Arthroplast 2018;33(7S):S76–80.
36. Cizmic Z, et al. Hip and knee section, prevention, host related: proceedings of international consensus on orthopedic infections. J Arthroplast. 2019;34(2S):S255–70.
37. Chong RW, Chong CS, Lai CH. Total hip arthroplasty in patients with chronic autoimmune inflammatory arthroplasties. Int J Rheum Dis. 2010;13(3):235–9.
38. Baker JF, George MD. Prevention of infection in the perioperative setting in patients with rheumatic disease treated with immunosuppression. Curr Rheumatol Rep. 2019;21(5):17.
39. Dimitriou D, et al. Human immunodeficiency virus infection and hip and knee arthroplasty. JBJS Rev. 2017;5(9):e8.
40. Falakassa J, Diaz A, Schneiderbauer M. Outcomes of total joint arthroplasty in HIV patients. Iowa Orthop J. 2014;34:102–6.
41. Jacob R, et al. Incidence of complications and revision surgery in HAART compliant HIV patients undergoing primary total hip and knee arthroplasty: an institutional review. Arch Orthop Trauma Surg. 2022;143:3803.
42. Charnley J. A clean-air operating enclosure. Br J Surg. 1964;51:202–5.
43. Tanner J, Woodings D, Moncaster K. Preoperative hair removal to reduce surgical site infection. Cochrane Database Syst Rev. 2006;2:CD004122.
44. Harrasser N, Harnoss T. [Prevention of periprosthetic joint infections]. Wien Med Wochenschr. 2012;162(5–6):115–20.
45. Jahoda D, et al. [Antibiotic treatment for prevention of infectious complications in joint replacement]. Acta Chir Orthop Traumatol Cechoslov. 2006;73(2):108–14.
46. Gyssens IC. Preventing postoperative infections: current treatment recommendations. Drugs. 1999;57(2):175–85.
47. Dellinger EP, et al. Quality standard for antimicrobial prophylaxis in surgical procedures. The Infectious Diseases Society of America. Infect Control Hosp Epidemiol. 1994;15(3):182–8.
48. Bratzler DW, et al. Antimicrobial prophylaxis for surgery: an advisory statement from the National Surgical Infection Prevention Project. Clin Infect Dis 2004;38(12):1706–15.
49. van Kasteren ME, et al. [Optimizing antibiotics policy in The Netherlands. V. SWAB guidelines for perioperative antibiotic prophylaxis. Foundation Antibiotics Policy Team]. Ned Tijdschr Geneeskd. 2000;144(43):2049–55.
50. Aboltins CA, et al. Hip and knee section, prevention, antimicrobials (systemic): proceedings of international consensus on orthopedic infections. J Arthroplast. 2019;34(2S):S279–88.
51. Wyles CC, et al. John Charnley award: increased risk of prosthetic joint infection following primary total knee and hip arthroplasty with the use of alternative antibiotics to cefazolin: the value of allergy testing for antibiotic prophylaxis. Bone Joint J. 2019;101-B(6 Suppl B):9–15.
52. Blumenthal KG, et al. The impact of a reported penicillin allergy on surgical site infection risk. Clin Infect Dis. 2018;66(3):329–36.
53. Rondon AJ, et al. Cefazolin prophylaxis for total joint arthroplasty: obese patients are frequently underdosed and at increased risk of periprosthetic joint infection. J Arthroplast. 2018;33(11):3551–4.

54. Vorobeichik L, Weber EA, Tarshis J. Misconceptions surrounding penicillin allergy: implications for anesthesiologists. Anesth Analg. 2018;127(3):642–9.
55. Campagna JD, et al. The use of cephalosporins in penicillin-allergic patients: a literature review. J Emerg Med. 2012;42(5):612–20.
56. Wade RG, et al. The comparative efficacy of chlorhexidine gluconate and povidone-iodine antiseptics for the prevention of infection in clean surgery: a systematic review and network meta-analysis. Ann Surg. 2021;274(6):e481–8.
57. Noorani A, et al. Systematic review and meta-analysis of preoperative antisepsis with chlorhexidine versus povidone-iodine in clean-contaminated surgery. Br J Surg. 2010;97(11):1614–20.
58. Azboy I, et al. General assembly, prevention, risk mitigation, general factors: proceedings of international consensus on orthopedic infections. J Arthroplast. 2019;34(2S):S55–9.
59. Parienti JJ, et al. Hand-rubbing with an aqueous alcoholic solution vs traditional surgical hand-scrubbing and 30-day surgical site infection rates: a randomized equivalence study. JAMA. 2002;288(6):722–7.
60. Markatos K, Kaseta M, Nikolaou VS. Perioperative skin preparation and draping in modern total joint arthroplasty: current evidence. Surg Infect. 2015;16(3):221–5.
61. Webster J, Alghamdi AA. Use of plastic adhesive drapes during surgery for preventing surgical site infection. Cochrane Database Syst Rev. 2007;4:CD006353.
62. Baykasoglu A, Dereli T, Yilankirkan N. Application of cost/benefit analysis for surgical gown and drape selection: a case study. Am J Infect Control. 2009;37(3):215–26.
63. Ricciardi BF, et al. Prevention of surgical site infection in total joint arthroplasty: an international tertiary care center survey. HSS J. 2014;10(1):45–51.
64. Baldini A, et al. General assembly, prevention, operating room—personnel: proceedings of international consensus on orthopedic infections. J Arthroplast. 2019;34(2S):S97–S104.
65. Russell M, et al. Is there a time-dependent contamination risk to open surgical trays during total hip and knee arthroplasty? Iowa Orthop J. 2022;42(2):107–11.
66. Ahmed SS, Haddad FS. Prosthetic joint infection. Bone Joint Res. 2019;8(11):570–2.
67. Furnes O, et al. Failure mechanisms after unicompartmental and tricompartmental primary knee replacement with cement. J Bone Joint Surg Am. 2007;89(3):519–25.
68. Dai WL, et al. Outcomes following revision total knee arthroplasty septic versus aseptic failure: a national propensity-score-matched comparison. J Knee Surg. 2021;34(11):1227–36.
69. Clesham K, et al. Second-site prosthetic joint infection in patients with multiple prosthetic joints. Eur J Orthop Surg Traumatol. 2018;28(7):1369–74.
70. Urquhart DM, et al. Incidence and risk factors for deep surgical site infection after primary total hip arthroplasty: a systematic review. J Arthroplast. 2010;25(8):1216–22.e1–3.
71. Scigliano NM, et al. Operative time and risk of surgical site infection and periprosthetic joint infection: a systematic review and meta-analysis. Iowa Orthop J. 2022;42(1):155–61.
72. Orland MD, et al. Surgical duration implicated in major postoperative complications in total hip and total knee arthroplasty: a retrospective cohort study. J Am Acad Orthop Surg Glob Res Rev. 2020;4(11):e2000043.
73. Naranje S, et al. Does operative time affect infection rate in primary total knee arthroplasty? Clin Orthop Relat Res. 2015;473(1):64–9.
74. Namdari S, et al. Primary total joint arthroplasty performed in operating rooms following cases of known infection. Orthopedics. 2011;34(9):e541–5.
75. Chang CC, et al. Anesthetic management and surgical site infections in total hip or knee replacement: a population-based study. Anesthesiology. 2010;113(2):279–84.
76. Forbes SS, McLean RF. Review article: the anesthesiologist's role in the prevention of surgical site infections. Can J Anaesth. 2013;60(2):176–83.
77. Turina M, Fry DE, Polk HC Jr. Acute hyperglycemia and the innate immune system: clinical, cellular, and molecular aspects. Crit Care Med. 2005;33(7):1624–33.
78. Serino J III, et al. General versus neuraxial anesthesia in revision surgery for periprosthetic joint infection. J Arthroplast. 2022;37(8S):S971–6.
79. Arnold WV, et al. General assembly, prevention, postoperative factors: proceedings of international consensus on orthopedic infections. J Arthroplast. 2019;34(2S):S169–74.

80. Saleh K, et al. Predictors of wound infection in hip and knee joint replacement: results from a 20 year surveillance program. J Orthop Res. 2002;20(3):506–15.
81. Patel VP, et al. Factors associated with prolonged wound drainage after primary total hip and knee arthroplasty. J Bone Joint Surg Am. 2007;89(1):33–8.
82. Olukoya O, Fultang J. Aspirin compared with other anticoagulants for use as venous thromboembolism prophylaxis in elective orthopaedic hip and knee operations: a narrative literature review. Cureus. 2021;13(9):e18249.
83. Garbedian S, Sternheim A, Backstein D. Wound healing problems in total knee arthroplasty. Orthopedics. 2011;34(9):e516–8.
84. Doran MF, et al. Frequency of infection in patients with rheumatoid arthritis compared with controls: a population-based study. Arthritis Rheum. 2002;46(9):2287–93.
85. Klement MR, et al. Tranexamic acid reduces the rate of periprosthetic joint infection after aseptic revision arthroplasty. J Bone Joint Surg Am. 2020;102(15):1344–50.
86. Sharqzad AS, et al. Blood loss and allogeneic transfusion for surgical treatment of periprosthetic joint infection: a comparison of one- vs. two-stage exchange total hip arthroplasty. Int Orthop. 2019;43(9):2025–30.
87. Akonjom M, et al. General assembly, prevention, blood conservation: proceedings of international consensus on orthopedic infections. J Arthroplast. 2019;34(2S):S147–55.
88. Okafor C, et al. Cost of septic and aseptic revision total knee arthroplasty: a systematic review. BMC Musculoskelet Disord. 2021;22(1):706.
89. Yayac M, et al. Orthopedic specialty hospitals are associated with lower rates of deep surgical site infection compared with tertiary medical centers. Orthopedics. 2021;44(4):e521–6.

Diagnosis of Periprosthetic Joint Infection

Saad Tarabichi and Javad Parvizi

Introduction

Periprosthetic joint infection (PJI) is one of the leading causes of implant failure following primary and revision total joint arthroplasty (TJA) [1, 2]. Recent estimates have placed the incidence of PJI between 0.5% and 2% after total knee arthroplasty (TKA) and 0.5% and 1% after total hip arthroplasty (THA) [3, 4]. Despite collaborative efforts, as the number of TJA procedures performed annually continues to rise, inevitably, the number of PJI cases is also expected to increase [5].

To date, we are yet to identify a single "gold-standard" test for the diagnosis of PJI. Physicians often rely on a combination of serological tests, synovial markers, and clinical judgment in the workup of patients with suspected PJI [6, 7]. Although advancements in technology have led to the identification of promising tests that have greatly improved diagnostic confidence, the diagnosis of PJI remains challenging, and can be difficult to make [8–10].

Regardless of the affected joint, the workup of patients with suspected PJI typically follows a stepwise approach. First, patients undergo venipuncture for analysis of inflammatory markers. If these tests return negative, and in the absence of additional signs, no further investigations are recommended [11]. The next step in the workup of patients with elevated serological markers is arthrocentesis and subsequent biomarker testing. In addition to this, culture is routinely performed on synovial fluid samples taken during joint aspirations [12–14].

S. Tarabichi (✉)
Rothman Orthopaedic Institute, Philadelphia, PA, USA
Department of Orthopaedic Surgery, Mayo Clinic, Scottsdale, AZ, USA
e-mail: Saad.Tarabichi@rothmanortho.com

J. Parvizi
International Joint Center, Acibadem University Hospital, Istanbul, Turkey

This chapter will serve as a brief overview of the different diagnostic modalities and proposed criteria currently available to aid in the diagnosis of this disease process.

Serological Tests

C-Reactive Protein and Erythrocyte Sedimentation Rate

As a result of their high sensitivity and widespread availability, serum C-reactive protein (CRP) and erythrocyte sedimentation rate (ESR) are commonly utilized to rule out PJI in patients presenting with a painful prosthesis [15, 16]. However, a growing body evidence has shown that CRP and ESR are non-specific and can be normal in cases of PJI caused by indolent organisms (Coagulase-negative *Staphylococci* and *Cutibacterium acnes*) [17, 18].

D-Dimer

D-dimer has long been recognized for its prognostic utility in the setting of bacteremia and sepsis [19, 20]. Although the diagnostic utility of D-dimer has since been demonstrated in the orthopedic literature, conflicting reports on its performance have prevented it from widespread adoption in this setting [21–25]. It is important to note that variability in protocols pertaining to the measurement of D-dimer levels may not allow for the implementation of a universal diagnostic threshold [26]. Hence, external validation of proposed cutoffs by individual institutions is recommended [27].

Synovial Fluid Markers

White Blood Cell Count and Polymorphonuclear Leukocyte Percentage

Synovial white blood cell (WBC) count and polymorphonuclear leukocyte percentage (PMN%) have both been shown to have high accuracy for the diagnosis of PJI [28–31]. In its most recent definition of PJI, the 2018 International Consensus Meeting (ICM) on musculoskeletal infection proposed diagnostic thresholds of 3000 cells/μL for WBC count and 80% for PMN% [32]. Using the aforementioned cutoffs, the authors of a subsequent study found that WBC count exhibited a sensitivity and specificity of 86% and 83%, respectively, while PMN% demonstrated a sensitivity and specificity of 86% and 81%, respectively, in the diagnosis of PJI [11].

Alpha Defensin

Although all synovial biomarkers have been shown to exhibit excellent accuracy for the diagnosis of PJI, a recent study suggested that alpha defensin may be superior to other markers commonly used in this setting [33–36]. However, this has since been disputed by the findings of two subsequent studies [37, 38]. Due to its high cost, limited availability, and longer turnaround time, compared to conventional synovial biomarkers, routine measurement of alpha defensin may be of little value.

Other Tests

Imaging

Over the years, advancements in technology have resulted in the widespread availability of several different imaging modalities [39]. Notwithstanding, it is well-established that radiographic findings from conventional plain film radiographs, magnetic resonance imaging, and three-phase bone scans are poorly sensitive for the diagnosis of PJI [40–47]. For example, a recent meta-analysis found that three-phase bone scans had a pooled sensitivity and specificity of 64% and 97%, respectively [48]. Thus, clinical practice guidelines (CPGs) do not recommend routine ordering of these tests in the workup of patients with suspected PJI [49].

IL-6 and Procalcitonin

Interlukin-6 (IL-6) is commonly secreted cytokine that can stimulate the liver to produce acute phase reactants that are responsible for inflammation [50, 51]. By contrast, procalcitonin, itself an acute phase reactant, originates from embryologic derivatives of neural crest cells [52]. Although both aforementioned markers have demonstrated promising reports in the orthopedic literature, the absence of a validated diagnostic threshold has precluded them from widespread adoption [53].

Pathology

In cases of diagnostic uncertainty, histopathologic examination of periprosthetic tissues to look for neutrophilic infiltration can be a useful tool and is commonly performed [54, 55]. However, recent improvements in the accuracy of preoperative testing have resulted in a decrease in reliance on this technique. Furthermore, interobserver reliability in this setting remains a significant concern [56].

Spectro Analysis

A growing body of evidence has demonstrated that mass spectrometry, a proven method of microbial identification, may be a useful tool for the diagnosis of PJI [57, 58]. In a recent study, the authors found that MS demonstrated an area under the curve (AUC) of 0.975 for identifying PJI [59]. However, due to its high cost and limited availability, spectro analysis is not currently part of the routine workup of patients with suspected PJI.

Pathogen Identification

Culture

Despite its well-established limitations, culture remains the "gold-standard" method of pathogen identification in patients with PJI [8]. Although a recent study found that culture had a sensitivity and specificity of 70% and 97%, respectively, for the diagnosis of PJI, the incidence of culture negative PJI has been shown to be on the rise [60, 61]. It is also important to note that cultures of synovial fluid obtained during arthrocentesis are not as reliable as previously believed and may not always identify the true infecting pathogen [62].

Molecular Techniques

The utilization of molecular techniques for pathogen identification has increased significantly in recent years [63, 64]. In contrast to traditional culture, molecular techniques detect microbial DNA and thus have very high sensitivity [65–67]. In particular, the diagnostic utility of multiplex polymerase chain reaction (PCR) and next-generation sequencing (NGS) has been repeatedly examined in the orthopedic literature [68, 69]. In a recent study, NGS was capable of identifying an organism in >65% of patients with culture negative PJI [70]. In addition to this, the high sensitivity and fast turnaround time of molecular techniques may allow for earlier administration of targeted antimicrobial therapy [71].

Diagnostic Criteria

2018 ICM Criteria

In 2018, the workgroup of the ICM on musculoskeletal infection put forth the first evidence-based and validated criteria for the definition of PJI [32]. Patients were categorized as infected if they had evidence of either one of the following major

Major criteria (at least one of the following)	Decision
Two positive cultures of the same organism	Infected
Sinus tract with evidence of communication to the joint or visualization of the prosthesis	

		Minor Criteria	Score	Decision
Preoperative Diagnosis	Serum	Elevated CRP *or* D-Dimer	2	≥6 Infected
		Elevated ESR	1	2-5 Possibly Infected [a]
	Synovial	Elevated synovial *WBC count or* LE	3	0-1 Not Infected
		Positive alpha-defensin	3	
		Elevated synovial PMN (%)	2	
		Elevated synovial CRP	1	

	Inconclusive pre-op score *or* dry tap [a]	Score	Decision
Intraoperative Diagnosis	Preoperative score	-	≥6 Infected
	Positive histology	3	4-5 Inconclusive [b]
	Positive purulence	3	≤3 Not Infected
	Single positive culture	2	

Reproduced with permission from the Journal of Arthroplasty, License number: 5402600689340

Fig. 1 2018 ICM criteria for the diagnosis of hip and knee periprosthetic joint infection. (*Reproduced with permission from the Journal of Arthroplasty, License number: 5402600689340*)

criteria: (1) presence of a sinus tract or (2) ≥2 positive cultures isolating the same organism. In addition to this, random forest analyses were performed in order to assign a score and weight to individual serological tests, synovial markers, intraoperative findings, and culture results. Consequently, a raw ICM score is applied, and patients are classified as infected (≥6), inconclusive (4 or 5), or aseptic (0–3) (Fig. 1).

EBJIS Criteria

The European bone and joint infection society (EBJIS) utilizes clinical signs, radiographic findings, and serological and synovial biomarkers to classify patients into three distinct groups: (1) infection unlikely, (2) infection likely, or (3) infection confirmed [72]. It is important to note that the EBJIS criteria classifies patients as infected based on the positivity of single synovial biomarkers, without considering the possibility of a false-positive result. Furthermore, the aforementioned diagnostic criteria have not been validated to date.

Summary

Although the development of several evidence-based criteria has significantly improved diagnostic confidence in this setting, the diagnosis of PJI can be challenging. This chapter provides the reader with a brief review of the different modalities currently available to aid in the diagnosis of PJI.

References

1. Namba RS, Inacio MCS, Paxton EW. Risk factors associated with deep surgical site infections after primary total knee arthroplasty: an analysis of 56,216 knees. J Bone Joint Surg Am. 2013;95:775–82. https://doi.org/10.2106/JBJS.L.00211.
2. Kurtz SM, Lau E, Watson H, Schmier JK, Parvizi J. Economic burden of periprosthetic joint infection in the United States. J Arthroplast. 2012;27:61–5.e1. https://doi.org/10.1016/j.arth.2012.02.022.
3. Edwards JR, Peterson KD, Mu Y, Banerjee S, Allen-Bridson K, Morrell G, et al. National Healthcare Safety Network (NHSN) report: data summary for 2006 through 2008, issued December 2009. Am J Infect Control. 2009;37:783–805. https://doi.org/10.1016/j.ajic.2009.10.001.
4. Sandiford NA, Franceschini M, Kendoff D. The burden of prosthetic joint infection (PJI). Ann Joint. 2021;6:25. https://doi.org/10.21037/aoj-2020-pji-11.
5. Springer BD, Cahue S, Etkin CD, Lewallen DG, McGrory BJ. Infection burden in total hip and knee arthroplasties: an international registry-based perspective. Arthroplast Today. 2017;3:137–40. https://doi.org/10.1016/j.artd.2017.05.003.
6. Wasterlain AS, Goswami K, Ghasemi SA, Parvizi J. Diagnosis of periprosthetic infection: recent developments. JBJS. 2020;102:1366–75. https://doi.org/10.2106/JBJS.19.00598.
7. Goh GS, Parvizi J. Diagnosis and treatment of culture-negative periprosthetic joint infection. J Arthroplast. 2022;37:1488. https://doi.org/10.1016/j.arth.2022.01.061.
8. Kim S-J, Cho YJ. Current guideline for diagnosis of periprosthetic joint infection: a review article. Hip Pelvis. 2021;33:11–7. https://doi.org/10.5371/hp.2021.33.1.11.
9. Bonanzinga T, Ferrari MC, Tanzi G, Vandenbulcke F, Zahar A, Marcacci M. The role of alpha defensin in prosthetic joint infection (PJI) diagnosis: a literature review. EFORT Open Rev. 2019;4:10–3. https://doi.org/10.1302/2058-5241.4.180029.
10. Alijanipour P, Bakhshi H, Parvizi J. Diagnosis of periprosthetic joint infection: the threshold for serological markers. Clin Orthop Relat Res. 2013;471:3186–95. https://doi.org/10.1007/s11999-013-3070-z.
11. Shahi A, Tan TL, Kheir MM, Tan DD, Parvizi J. Diagnosing periprosthetic joint infection: and the winner is? J Arthroplast. 2017;32:S232–5. https://doi.org/10.1016/j.arth.2017.06.005.
12. Patel R, Osmon DR, Hanssen AD. The diagnosis of prosthetic joint infection: current techniques and emerging technologies. Clin Orthop Relat Res 2005;(437):55–8. https://doi.org/10.1097/01.blo.0000175121.73675.fd.
13. Parvizi J, Ghanem E, Sharkey P, Aggarwal A, Burnett RSJ, Barrack RL. Diagnosis of infected total knee: findings of a multicenter database. Clin Orthop Relat Res. 2008;466:2628–33. https://doi.org/10.1007/s11999-008-0471-5.
14. Parvizi J, Fassihi SC, Enayatollahi MA. Diagnosis of periprosthetic joint infection following hip and knee arthroplasty. Orthop Clin North Am. 2016;47:505–15. https://doi.org/10.1016/j.ocl.2016.03.001.
15. Bingham JS, Hassebrock JD, Christensen AL, Beauchamp CP, Clarke HD, Spangehl MJ. Screening for periprosthetic joint infections with ESR and CRP: the ideal cutoffs. J Arthroplast. 2020;35:1351–4. https://doi.org/10.1016/j.arth.2019.11.040.

16. Austin MS, Ghanem E, Joshi A, Lindsay A, Parvizi J. A simple, cost-effective screening protocol to rule out periprosthetic infection. J Arthroplast. 2008;23:65–8. https://doi.org/10.1016/j.arth.2007.09.005.
17. Kheir MM, Tan TL, Shohat N, Foltz C, Parvizi J. Routine diagnostic tests for periprosthetic joint infection demonstrate a high false-negative rate and are influenced by the infecting organism. JBJS. 2018;100:2057–65. https://doi.org/10.2106/JBJS.17.01429.
18. Kanafani ZA, Sexton DJ, Pien BC, Varkey J, Basmania C, Kaye KS. Postoperative joint infections due to Propionibacterium species: a case-control study. Clin Infect Dis. 2009;49:1083–5. https://doi.org/10.1086/605577.
19. Meini S, Sozio E, Bertolino G, Sbrana F, Ripoli A, Pallotto C, et al. D-dimer as biomarker for early prediction of clinical outcomes in patients with severe invasive infections due to Streptococcus Pneumoniae and Neisseria Meningitidis. Front Med. 2021;8:627830.
20. Han Y-Q, Yan L, Zhang L, Ouyang P-H, Li P, Lippi G, et al. Performance of D-dimer for predicting sepsis mortality in the intensive care unit. Biochem Med (Zagreb). 2021;31:020709. https://doi.org/10.11613/BM.2021.020709.
21. Shahi A, Kheir MM, Tarabichi M, Hosseinzadeh HRS, Tan TL, Parvizi J. Serum D-dimer test is promising for the diagnosis of periprosthetic joint infection and timing of reimplantation. J Bone Joint Surg Am. 2017;99:1419–27. https://doi.org/10.2106/JBJS.16.01395.
22. Muñoz-Mahamud E, Tornero E, Estrada JA, Fernández-Valencia JA, Martínez-Pastor JC, Soriano Á. Usefulness of serum D-dimer and platelet count to mean platelet volume ratio to rule out chronic periprosthetic joint infection. J Bone Joint Infect. 2022;7:109–15. https://doi.org/10.5194/jbji-7-109-2022.
23. Wang R, Zhang H, Ding P, Jiao Q. The accuracy of D-dimer in the diagnosis of periprosthetic infections: a systematic review and meta-analysis. J Orthop Surg Res. 2022;17:99. https://doi.org/10.1186/s13018-022-03001-y.
24. Pan L, Wu H, Liu H, Yang X, Meng Z, Cao Y. Fibrinogen performs better than D-dimer for the diagnosis of periprosthetic joint infection: a meta-analysis of diagnostic trials. J Orthop Surg Res. 2021;16:30. https://doi.org/10.1186/s13018-020-02109-3.
25. Ackmann T, Möllenbeck B, Gosheger G, Schwarze J, Schmidt-Braekling T, Schneider KN, et al. Comparing the diagnostic value of serum D-dimer to CRP and IL-6 in the diagnosis of chronic prosthetic joint infection. J Clin Med. 2020;9:2917. https://doi.org/10.3390/jcm9092917.
26. Riley RS, Gilbert AR, Dalton JB, Pai S, McPherson RA. Widely used types and clinical applications of D-dimer assay. Lab Med. 2016;47:90–102. https://doi.org/10.1093/labmed/lmw001.
27. Pearson LN, Moser KA, Schmidt RL. D-dimer varies widely across instrument platforms and is not a reliable indicator of periprosthetic joint infections. Arthroplast Today. 2020;6:686–8. https://doi.org/10.1016/j.artd.2020.07.014.
28. Mason JB, Fehring TK, Odum SM, Griffin WL, Nussman DS. The value of white blood cell counts before revision total knee arthroplasty. J Arthroplast. 2003;18:1038–43. https://doi.org/10.1016/s0883-5403(03)00448-0.
29. Trampuz A, Hanssen AD, Osmon DR, Mandrekar J, Steckelberg JM, Patel R. Synovial fluid leukocyte count and differential for the diagnosis of prosthetic knee infection. Am J Med. 2004;117:556–62. https://doi.org/10.1016/j.amjmed.2004.06.022.
30. Bedair H, Ting N, Jacovides C, Saxena A, Moric M, Parvizi J, et al. The Mark Coventry Award: diagnosis of early postoperative TKA infection using synovial fluid analysis. Clin Orthop Relat Res. 2011;469:34–40. https://doi.org/10.1007/s11999-010-1433-2.
31. Dinneen A, Guyot A, Clements J, Bradley N. Synovial fluid white cell and differential count in the diagnosis or exclusion of prosthetic joint infection. Bone Joint J. 2013;95-B:554–7. https://doi.org/10.1302/0301-620X.95B4.30388.
32. Parvizi J, Tan TL, Goswami K, Higuera C, Valle CD, Chen AF, et al. The 2018 definition of periprosthetic hip and knee infection: an evidence-based and validated criteria. J Arthroplast. 2018;33:1309–1314.e2. https://doi.org/10.1016/j.arth.2018.02.078.

33. Lee YS, Koo K-H, Kim HJ, Tian S, Kim T-Y, Maltenfort MG, et al. Synovial fluid biomarkers for the diagnosis of periprosthetic joint infection: a systematic review and meta-analysis. J Bone Joint Surg Am. 2017;99:2077–84. https://doi.org/10.2106/JBJS.17.00123.
34. Parvizi J, Jacovides C, Antoci V, Ghanem E. Diagnosis of periprosthetic joint infection: the utility of a simple yet unappreciated enzyme. JBJS. 2011;93:2242–8. https://doi.org/10.2106/JBJS.J.01413.
35. Deirmengian C, Kardos K, Kilmartin P, Cameron A, Schiller K, Parvizi J. Diagnosing periprosthetic joint infection: has the era of the biomarker arrived? Clin Orthop Relat Res. 2014;472:3254–62. https://doi.org/10.1007/s11999-014-3543-8.
36. Frangiamore SJ, Gajewski ND, Saleh A, Farias-Kovac M, Barsoum WK, Higuera CA. α-Defensin accuracy to diagnose periprosthetic joint infection-best available test? J Arthroplast. 2016;31:456–60. https://doi.org/10.1016/j.arth.2015.09.035.
37. Kleeman-Forsthuber LT, Johnson RM, Brady AC, Pollet AK, Dennis DA, Jennings JM. Alpha-defensin offers limited utility in routine workup of periprosthetic joint infection. J Arthroplast. 2021;36:1746–52. https://doi.org/10.1016/j.arth.2020.12.018.
38. Ivy MI, Sharma K, Greenwood-Quaintance KE, Tande AJ, Osmon DR, Berbari EF, et al. Synovial fluid α defensin has comparable accuracy to synovial fluid white blood cell count and polymorphonuclear percentage for periprosthetic joint infection diagnosis. Bone Joint J. 2021;103-B:1119–26. https://doi.org/10.1302/0301-620X.103B6.BJJ-2020-1741.R1.
39. Smith-Bindman R, Miglioretti DL, Larson EB. Rising use of diagnostic medical imaging in a large integrated health system. Health Aff (Millwood). 2008;27:1491–502. https://doi.org/10.1377/hlthaff.27.6.1491.
40. Zajonz D, Wuthe L, Tiepolt S, Brandmeier P, Prietzel T, von Salis-Soglio GF, et al. Diagnostic work-up strategy for periprosthetic joint infections after total hip and knee arthroplasty: a 12-year experience on 320 consecutive cases. Patient Saf Surg. 2015;9:20. https://doi.org/10.1186/s13037-015-0071-8.
41. Lyons CW, Berquist TH, Lyons JC, Rand JA, Brown ML. Evaluation of radiographic findings in painful hip arthroplasties. Clin Orthop Relat Res. 1985;195:239–51.
42. Gelman MI, Coleman RE, Stevens PM, Davey BW. Radiography, radionuclide imaging, and arthrography in the evaluation of total hip and knee replacement. Radiology. 1978;128:677–82. https://doi.org/10.1148/128.3.677.
43. Weiss PE, Mall JC, Hoffer PB, Murray WR, Rodrigo JJ, Genant HK. 99mTc-methylene diphosphonate bone imaging in the evaluation of total hip prostheses. Radiology. 1979;133:727–9. https://doi.org/10.1148/133.3.727.
44. Glaudemans AWJM, Galli F, Pacilio M, Signore A. Leukocyte and bacteria imaging in prosthetic joint infection. Eur Cell Mater. 2013;25:61–77. https://doi.org/10.22203/ecm.v025a05.
45. Koch K, Lorbiecki J, Hinks S, King K. A multispectral three-dimensional technique for imaging near metal implants. Magn Reson Med. 2009;61:381–90. https://doi.org/10.1002/mrm.21856.
46. Hayter CL, Koff MF, Shah P, Koch KM, Miller TT, Potter HG. MRI after arthroplasty: comparison of MAVRIC and conventional fast spin-echo techniques. AJR Am J Roentgenol. 2011;197:W405–11. https://doi.org/10.2214/AJR.11.6659.
47. Hayter CL, Koff M, Perino G, Nawabi DH, Profile S, Hayter CL, et al. MRI findings in painful metal-on-metal hip arthroplasty. AJR Am J Roentgenol. 2012;199(4):884–93.
48. Figa R, Veloso M, Bernaus M, Ysamat M, González JM, Gómez L, et al. Should scintigraphy be completely excluded from the diagnosis of periprosthetic joint infection? Clin Radiol. 2020;75:797.e1–7. https://doi.org/10.1016/j.crad.2020.06.014.
49. Diaz C, Glaudemans A, Llinás A. What is the role of nuclear medicine imaging modalities (three-phase bone scintigraphy, bone marrow scintigraphy, white blood cell (WBC) scintigraphy [with 99mTc or 111In], anti-granulocyte monoclonal antibody scintigraphy and fluorodeoxyglucose-positron emission tomography/computed tomography (FDG-PET/CT) scan in diagnosing periprosthetic joint infection (PJI)? n.d.:2.
50. Barton BE. IL-6: insights into novel biological activities. Clin Immunol Immunopathol. 1997;85:16–20. https://doi.org/10.1006/clin.1997.4420.

51. Selberg O, Hecker H, Martin M, Klos A, Bautsch W, Köhl J. Discrimination of sepsis and systemic inflammatory response syndrome by determination of circulating plasma concentrations of procalcitonin, protein complement 3a, and interleukin-6. Crit Care Med. 2000;28:2793–8. https://doi.org/10.1097/00003246-200008000-00019.
52. Xie K, Qu X, Yan M. Procalcitonin and α-defensin for diagnosis of periprosthetic joint infections. J Arthroplast. 2017;32:1387–94. https://doi.org/10.1016/j.arth.2016.10.001.
53. Yoon J-R, Yang S-H, Shin Y-S. Diagnostic accuracy of interleukin-6 and procalcitonin in patients with periprosthetic joint infection: a systematic review and meta-analysis. Int Orthop. 2018;42:1213–26. https://doi.org/10.1007/s00264-017-3744-3.
54. Bémer P, Léger J, Milin S, Plouzeau C, Valentin AS, Stock N, et al. Histopathological diagnosis of prosthetic joint infection: does a threshold of 23 neutrophils do better than classification of the periprosthetic membrane in a prospective multicenter study? J Clin Microbiol. 2018;56:e00536-18. https://doi.org/10.1128/JCM.00536-18.
55. Bori G, McNally MA, Athanasou N. Histopathology in periprosthetic joint infection: when will the morphomolecular diagnosis be a reality? Biomed Res Int. 2018;2018:1412701. https://doi.org/10.1155/2018/1412701.
56. Goswami K, Parvizi J, Maxwell CP. Current recommendations for the diagnosis of acute and chronic PJI for hip and knee-cell counts, alpha-defensin, leukocyte esterase, next-generation sequencing. Curr Rev Musculoskelet Med. 2018;11:428–38. https://doi.org/10.1007/s12178-018-9513-0.
57. Patel R, Alijanipour P, Parvizi J. Advancements in diagnosing periprosthetic joint infections after total hip and knee arthroplasty. Open Orthop J. 2016;10:654–61. https://doi.org/10.2174/1874325001610010654.
58. Fox A. Mass spectrometry for species or strain identification after culture or without culture: past, present, and future. J Clin Microbiol. 2006;44:2677–80. https://doi.org/10.1128/JCM.00971-06.
59. Li R, Song L, Quan Q, Liu M-W, Chai W, Lu Q, et al. Detecting periprosthetic joint infection by using mass spectrometry. J Bone Joint Surg Am. 2021;103:1917–26. https://doi.org/10.2106/JBJS.20.01944.
60. Li C, Ojeda-Thies C, Trampuz A. Culture of periprosthetic tissue in blood culture bottles for diagnosing periprosthetic joint infection. BMC Musculoskelet Disord. 2019;20:299. https://doi.org/10.1186/s12891-019-2683-0.
61. Palan J, Nolan C, Sarantos K, Westerman R, King R, Foguet P. Culture-negative periprosthetic joint infections. EFORT Open Rev. 2019;4:585–94. https://doi.org/10.1302/2058-5241.4.180067.
62. Declercq P, Neyt J, Depypere M, Goris S, Van Wijngaerden E, Verhaegen J, et al. Preoperative joint aspiration culture results and causative pathogens in total hip and knee prosthesis infections: mind the gap. Acta Clin Belg. 2020;75:284–92. https://doi.org/10.1080/17843286.2019.1611718.
63. Ramamurthy T, Ghosh A, Pazhani GP, Shinoda S. Current perspectives on viable but non-culturable (VBNC) pathogenic bacteria. Front Public Health. 2014;2:103. https://doi.org/10.3389/fpubh.2014.00103.
64. Weile J, Knabbe C. Current applications and future trends of molecular diagnostics in clinical bacteriology. Anal Bioanal Chem. 2009;394:731–42. https://doi.org/10.1007/s00216-009-2779-8.
65. Tsui CKM, Woodhall J, Chen W, Lévesque CA, Lau A, Schoen CD, et al. Molecular techniques for pathogen identification and fungus detection in the environment. IMA Fungus. 2011;2:177–89. https://doi.org/10.5598/imafungus.2011.02.02.09.
66. Sigmund IK, Holinka J, Sevelda F, Staats K, Heisinger S, Kubista B, et al. Performance of automated multiplex polymerase chain reaction (mPCR) using synovial fluid in the diagnosis of native joint septic arthritis in adults. Bone Joint J. 2019;101-B:288–96. https://doi.org/10.1302/0301-620X.101B3.BJJ-2018-0868.R1.

67. Achermann Y, Vogt M, Leunig M, Wüst J, Trampuz A. Improved diagnosis of periprosthetic joint infection by multiplex PCR of sonication fluid from removed implants. J Clin Microbiol. 2010;48:1208–14. https://doi.org/10.1128/JCM.00006-10.
68. Tarabichi M, Alvand A, Shohat N, Goswami K, Parvizi J. Diagnosis of Streptococcus canis periprosthetic joint infection: the utility of next-generation sequencing. Arthroplast Today. 2018;4:20–3. https://doi.org/10.1016/j.artd.2017.08.005.
69. Tarabichi M, Shohat N, Goswami K, Parvizi J. Can next generation sequencing play a role in detecting pathogens in synovial fluid? Bone Joint J. 2018;100-B:127–33. https://doi.org/10.1302/0301-620X.100B2.BJJ-2017-0531.R2.
70. Goswami K, Clarkson S, Phillips CD, Dennis DA, Klatt BA, O'Malley MJ, et al. An enhanced understanding of culture-negative periprosthetic joint infection with next-generation sequencing: a multicenter study. J Bone Joint Surg Am. 2022;104:1523. https://doi.org/10.2106/JBJS.21.01061.
71. Tarabichi M, Shohat N, Goswami K, Alvand A, Silibovsky R, Belden K, et al. Diagnosis of periprosthetic joint infection: the potential of next-generation sequencing. J Bone Joint Surg Am. 2018;100:147–54. https://doi.org/10.2106/JBJS.17.00434.
72. McNally M, Sousa R, Wouthuyzen-Bakker M, Chen AF, Soriano A, Vogely HC, et al. The EBJIS definition of periprosthetic joint infection. Bone Joint J. 2021;103-B:18–25. https://doi.org/10.1302/0301-620X.103B1.BJJ-2020-1381.R1.

Multidisciplinary Team Management of Periprosthetic Knee Infections

Dia Eldean Giebaly, Andreas Fontalis, and Fares S. Haddad

Introduction

Prosthetic joint infection is a serious and devastating complication following arthroplasty and poses significant challenges for the patient, health care providers, and the treating institution. Despite an increasing understanding of the condition and the major preventive efforts put into patient related and surgical factors [1, 2], the incidence of PJI following hip or knee arthroplasty is reported to be 1–2% [1, 3], and infection is the main indication recorded in approximately 80% of either stage one or stage two procedures in the national joint registry [4]. In some units the infection rate is reported to be as high as 5% [5].

The volume of knee arthroplasty is increasing annually, and as such the revision burden will inevitably increase [6, 7]. It is projected that the number of revision procedures will increase dramatically over the coming 10 years [6, 8]. Not only is the number of revision procedures rising, but their associated costs are also increasing. The mean cost of revision treatment for an infected knee arthroplasty is quoted as three-times the cost of treatment for an aseptic knee at £30,000 [9, 10], with the cost of some procedures reaching in excess of £75,000 per patient [10].

Patients with prosthetic joint infections are challenging to diagnose and manage, they are often frail and elderly, with multiple comorbidities any may present acutely, often as emergencies or via referrals from neighboring hospitals. Acute management can be much more variable and is dependent on the stability of the patient,

D. E. Giebaly · A. Fontalis · F. S. Haddad (✉)
University College London Hospitals (UCLH), London, UK
e-mail: dia.giebaly@doctors.org.uk; andreas.fontalis@nhs.net; fsh@fareshaddad.net

© The Author(s), under exclusive license to Springer Nature Switzerland AG 2024
M. Citak et al. (eds.), *One-Stage Septic Revision Arthroplasty*,
https://doi.org/10.1007/978-3-031-59160-0_4

duration of symptoms, medical and immune status of the patient, local soft tissue factors, and virulence of the organism grown. Treatment options range from open irrigation and debridement and exchange of modular components to revision of the prosthesis via either a one- or two-stage revision arthroplasty.

A single-stage or two-stage revision has long been considered the "gold standard" for treating periprosthetic infections of the knee. Recent studies for one- and two-stage revision arthroplasty have shown similar results with success rates ranging from 72% to 100% [11–19]. However, retention of the prosthesis with irrigation and debridement and exchange of modular components followed by appropriate medical management remains a viable option for the acutely infected knee if performed in a thorough manner, under the correct circumstances and with significant expertise.

These patients may require multiple procedures and interventions, often presenting with confounding factors such as bone loss, joint instability, and deformity, and may require close monitoring both medically and surgically between interventions. These patients require technically more complex surgery [20] with a longer operating time, greater blood loss, and a higher rate of complications [21–25]. This leads to an increased length of stay, morbidity, and increased mortality compared with that experienced by patients undergoing primary TKA [10, 26]. Therefore, revision knee surgery, for any reason, is associated with increased costs.

Complex antibiotic plans for prolonged durations are frequently used that must adapt to the clinical situation, resistance of bacterial strains [27], as well as observing for side effects [1]. Long-term monitoring is also required after successful treatment to ensure that infection does not recur. Recurrence of the infection is high and reported between 8% and 70% [28, 29] and complications associated with surgery are common and carry high risks of morbidly and mortality [30, 31].

Therefore, the management of prosthetic joint infections must involve close liaison between different teams including orthopedic surgeons, microbiologists, infectious diseases specialists, plastic surgeons, nurses, and physiotherapists. Although in recent years steps have been made to provide pathways and guidance for individuals with a periprosthetic joint infection (PJI), there remains a lack of evidence and therefore consensus across many facets of patient care [10]. This may partly explain the variability of success rates in revision surgery for PJI across the literature [10, 32, 33].

Managing this increased volume and complexity of patients and increased associated costs requires a robust efficient approach to managing such cases. This usually requires input from various medical and surgical staff, nursing, and other specialist care in often changing and challenging situations and usually requires high level decision-making at multiple time points throughout the patient "journey."

The idea of the Knee Infection Multidisciplinary Team (MDT) was developed to ensure regular, adaptable, efficient care with the key decision makers using evidence-based principles [34]. MDTs bring together staff with the necessary knowledge, skills, and experience to ensure high quality diagnosis, treatment, and care [35–42]. However, this has not been well studied in the context of prosthetic joint infections.

Although there are promising results in the literature regarding the usage of a multidisciplinary team (MDT) for the treatment of PJI in prosthetic hips [33, 43–45], there is limited evidence available for the effectiveness of an MDT in the management of infected knees [44, 46]. We present in this chapter some of the related literature surrounding the use of MDT in PJI, the roles of different members within the MDT, challenges in setting up an MDT and some characteristics of a well-functioning service.

Literature Review

There is limited evidence available for the effectiveness of an MDT in the management of infected knee arthroplasty [44, 46, 47]. Here we present all the results of recent studies examining the results of managing PJI infections of both hip and knee arthroplasty.

Ibrahim et al. [33] reviewed 125 consecutive patients who underwent two-stage revision THA involving a multidisciplinary team approach between 2000 and 2008 by a single surgeon at a tertiary center with a mean follow-up was 8.6 years. The data were retrieved from a prospectively compiled database. Single-stage revision THA were excluded. The multidisciplinary team included microbiologists, infectious disease specialists, orthopedic surgeons, radiologists, physiotherapists, and physicians who reviewed all patients, and their management was discussed at every stage in their pathway. All patients included in this study satisfied the criteria for diagnosing periprosthetic joint infection as proposed by the American Musculoskeletal Infection Society [48–50]. They reported excellent control of infection supported by their multidisciplinary approach with a 96% control of infection at 5 years [33].

Ntalos et al. [45] examined the effectiveness of using a multidisciplinary conference discussed PJI, osteomyelitis, soft tissue infections, and osteosynthesis associated infections as part of their conference. Their retrospective review of PJI patients were divided into 2 groups, prior to ($n = 20$) then after to initiation of their conference ($n = 26$). A total of 46 patients were identified consisting of 12 infected hemiarthroplasties and 34 total hip arthroplasties. They organized weekly conferences, comprising of three specialties need to take part to validate multidisciplinary decision-making: a senior orthopedic surgeon, a senior pathologist, and a senior microbiologist were present. Each case was furthermore discussed with a senior radiologist. Patients discussed in the multidisciplinary conference showed a significantly shorter in-hospital stay (29 days vs. 62 days; $p < 0.05$), a significant reduction in procedures (1.8 vs. 5.2; $p < 0.05$), and a significant reduction in the requirement for antibiotics.

Without conference discussion, the favored procedure was debridement, antibiotics, and implant retention (DAIR) (9/20, 45%), whereas following conference consensus most patients were either treated with the one-stage (9/26, 35%) or two-stage exchange (8/26, 31%), followed by DAIR (7/26, 27%). In contrast, with the single discipline approach prior to multidisciplinary conference introduction, one- and two-stage strategy were performed in 15% and 25% retrospectively.

Akgun et al. [43] in their single-center prospective cohort study, all patients with hip PJI from March 2013 to May 2015 were treated using a standardized comprehensive diagnostic algorithm and two-stage exchange. Treatment failure was assessed according to the Delphi-based consensus definition and patients were followed up at a mean follow-up of 33.1 months. Individualized decision-making through a multidisciplinary team, including infectious disease specialists, internal medicine specialists, and orthopedic surgeons, who were involved in every stage of PJI management for each patient. The Kaplan-Meier estimated infection-free survival after 3 years was 89.3% (95% CI, 80–94%) with 30 patients at risk. The mean follow-up was 33.1 months (range, 24–48 months) with successful treatment of PJI [43].

Vuorinen et al. [46] in their retrospective series of patients examined the effectiveness of their multidisciplinary team in treatment of knee and hip PJI. Their study consisted of a total of 154 post-operative PJIs from 3 time periods, 21 PJIs from 2005 to 2007 (Group 1: prior to implementation of the MDT in 3 hospitals), 65 PJIs from 2011 to 2013 (Group 2: introduction of MDT and centralization of treatment in 1 hospital), and 68 PJIs from 2015 to 2016 (Group 3: Introduction of implant sonication and dedicated microbial sampling instrumentation) (Table 1). The multidisciplinary team included orthopedic surgeons, an infectious disease specialist working in close cooperation with a microbiology laboratory, and a plastic surgeon is available if needed [46].

During their study period, the use of DAIR as primary surgical treatment increased from 43% to 90%, and, simultaneously, the number of two-stage exchanges performed decreased from 52% to 16%. This change in treatment methods led to a decrease from 2 to 1 in the median number of operations per PJI. Additionally, there was a decrease of 65% in the median LOS [from 49.0 days (group 1) to 17 dts (group 3)] after the multidisciplinary team was established in their clinic. The successful outcome of DAIR improved from 55.6% (5/9, Group 1) to 85.2% (52/61, Group 3).

Biddle et al. [44] in their retrospective analysis from a single center compared 29 consecutive joints prior to and then after the implementation of an infection MDT. They showed that there was a significant difference in failure rates between the 2 groups with 12 patients (41.38%) prior to the MDT requiring further revision surgery compared to only on patient (6.67%) after implementation of their MDT. Their MDT included a consultant microbiologist, a consultant in infectious diseases, along with several orthopedic consultants with an interest in PJI and revision surgery [44]. They have now also included a pharmacist to their MDT. The team would meet routinely once a week for face-to-face discussions. Notes from the MDT were uploaded to online patient archives.

Razi et al. [47] described the results of their Cardiff experience in 84 patients undergoing single-stage revision for infected total knee arthroplasty. They used a standardized debridement protocol and multidisciplinary input with relatively broad selection criteria. Patients were not excluded for culture negative PJI or the presence of a sinus. A total of 76 patients (90.5%) were infection-free at a mean follow-up of 7 years, with 8 reinfections (9.5%). Culture negative PJI was not associated with a higher reinfection rate ($p = 0.343$). However, there was a significantly higher rate of

Table 1 Results of reported studies utilizing a multidisciplinary team approach in treatment of PJI of the hip and knee

Author, date	Patient cohort	Study type	Outcomes	Key results	Study weakness
Ibrahim et al. [33] 2014	– 125 patients – Two-stage revision – THA	Retrospective (level IV evidence)	– Rate of control of infection at 5 years – Harris hip score (HHS)	– 96% control of infection at 5 years – The mean HHS was 38 pre-operatively and had improved to 81.2 at 5 years	– 19 patients died but not related to PJI – Single surgeon series
Ntalos et al. [45] 2018	– 46 patients in total (12 infected hemiarthroplasties and 34 THA) – 26 discussed in MDT vs. 20 prior to MDT	Retrospective (level IV evidence)	– Length of stay – Number of surgical procedures – Total number of applied antibiotics	– Significantly shorter in-hospital stay (29 vs. 62 days; $p < 0.05$) – Significant reduction in total surgical procedures (1.8 vs. 5.1; $p < 0.05$)	– Retrospective – Lack of randomization – Small number of patients – Total time course of applied antibiotics not fully available for analysis – Different treatment modalities between the two groups
Akgun et al. [43] 2019	– 84 patients in total – THA – Two-stage revision	Prospective (level IV evidence)	– Infection-free survival	– The Kaplan-Meier estimated infection-free survival after 3 years was 89.3%	– Observational study from single center – Short follow-up at 33 months
Vuorinen et al. [46] 2021	– 154 patients in total – Knee and hip revisions – 3 groups – Group 1 ($n = 21$) – Group 2 ($n = 65$) – Group 3 ($n = 68$)	Retrospective (level IV evidence)	– Length of stay – Number and type of surgical procedures – Antibiotic duration	– Median number of operations decreased from 2 to 1 procedure – Median LOS decreased from 49 days to 17 days – Improved success with DAIR	– Retrospective – Diagnosis of PJI disorganized and treated at three hospitals – Goal at the end of study period shifted to single-stage treatment and therefore shorter antibiotic duration

(continued)

Table 1 (continued)

Author, date	Patient cohort	Study type	Outcomes	Key results	Study weakness
Biddle et al. [44] 2021	– 29 consecutive patients (15 knees, 14 hips) pre-MDT vs. 29 consecutive patients post-MDT (15 knees, 14 hips)	Retrospective (level IV evidence)	– Successfully treated PJI based on Delphi international multidisciplinary consensus [51]	– There was a significant difference in failure rates between the two groups ($p = 0.001$, Fisher's exact test) – 12 individuals (41.38%) pre-MDT requiring further surgery compared with one individual (6.67%) post-MDT	– Retrospective – Minimum 2 years follow-up – Single unit with several revision surgeons performing the procedures – Plans prior to implementation of the MDT was up to the discretion of each surgeon
Razi et al. [47] 2021	– 84 patients in total – 37 patients with infected primary TKA – 47 patients with infected TKA revisions – All treated with single-stage revision TKA	Retrospective (level IV evidence)	– Successfully treated PJU – Reinfection – PROMS (OKS)	– 76 patients (90.5%) infection free at 7 years post operatively – Culture negative PJI was not associated with a higher infection rate	– Retrospective – Cohort heterogenous group of organisms and host factors

recurrence in patients with polymicrobial infections ($p = 0.003$). They concluded one-stage exchange, using a strict debridement protocol and multidisciplinary input, is an effective treatment option for the infected TKA.

What Comprises an MDT?

Most of the literature describing the multidisciplinary approach has stemmed from cancer services [37–39, 41, 42, 52, 53] where this has become the established pathway of care. Limited published studies examining the benefits of MDT's have focused on clinical results after PJI of the hips and knee arthroplasty [33, 43–47, 54]. Important principle of care delivery in this setting is consideration of the wholistic needs of the patient and including appropriate specialists to address these issues. In the context of PJI the following team members are required:

Orthopaedic and Plastic Surgeons

Most commonly the MDT is led by the orthopedic surgeon who orchestrates and encourages a multidisciplinary approach. While the decision regarding the type and timing of the operation ultimately lies with the surgeon, infection specialists can provide vital information to inform decision-making. It is therefore imperative to approach the MDT with an open mind and employ a patient-centered approach. The MDT meetings should be held regularly (e.g., on a weekly basis) either face-to-face or online and the Orthopedic Consultant in charge should have a special interest in PJI and revision surgery. It is recommended that they should be fellowship trained in revision arthroplasty surgery and/or have considerable experience in high volume centers treating patients with PJI.

The presence of a Consultant Plastic Surgeon with a special interest in lower limb reconstruction surgery is also desirable, particularly when soft tissue coverage or post-operative soft tissue management is anticipated to be challenging.

Microbiologist

Undoubtedly, the role of the microbiologist or infection specialist is vital to the MDT. Their involvement begins with ensuring the diagnosis of PJI is established. This is particularly important in case of culture negative PJI, when operative findings of infection (e.g., presence of sinus or purulent discharge from the joint) are present.

Another important component of the MDT that should not be overlooked is a root cause analysis. This presents the opportunity to identify case specific challenges and better understand the complexity of the risk factors involved. Hereto, the expert and specialist knowledge of the infection specialist pertaining to microbial metabolism, prevalence, methods of transmission, and host specific factors is essential. The analysis should encompass patient-specific risk factors and is pivotal to mitigate the risk for the arthroplasty service. Examples include the hematogenous spread of *Staphylococcus aureus* from an infected line, endocarditis, gram-negative bacilli that may indicate renal or gastrointestinal pathology or polymicrobial infection [55].

The specialist knowledge of antibiotic function, pharmacokinetics, and metabolism is essential to guide antibiotic management, which will be collectively decided with the orthopedic surgeon taking into consideration the clinical examination or intra-operative findings. Decision-making will also be guided by the virulence of specific organisms and the documented success rates of DAIR. Finally, there has been an evolution in the field of musculoskeletal microbiology which has led to significant findings and improvement to the antibiotic management of PJI patients as evidenced by the results of the OVIVA trial (Oral versus Intravenous Antibiotics for Bone and Joint Infection) [56, 57]. Therefore, it is important for the microbiologist involved to have a specialist musculoskeletal interest and work within a dedicated, musculoskeletal microbiology service [58].

Musculoskeletal Radiologist

Musculoskeletal radiologists play a central role in decision-making and should be an integral part of the multidisciplinary team. They provide specialist advice in relation to imaging modalities and interpretation of radiological findings. Their input is particularly important in subtle case, where contextualization of radiological signs is key.

Pharmacist

The involvement of pharmacists in MDT is also very important. Through their involvement with the day-to-day care of the PJI patient they will ensure appropriate drug monitoring and documentation of treatment. Furthermore, they will also liaise with outpatient services and ensure the smooth and timely supply of complex antibiotics in the community.

Nutritionist

Malnutrition is a well-documented prognostic factor for impaired wound healing and surgical infections. It also comprises an independent prognostic factor for chronic aseptic failure and acute post-operative infections [59, 60].

To that end, the expert knowledge of a nutritionist should complement the MDT meeting. Through specific nutritional screening tools and laboratory tests, such as albumin levels, lymphocyte count, glucose; they will identify the need for pre- and/or post-operative optimization of the nutritional status. Following risk stratification, they will also suggest a patient-tailored nutritional support, that will help reduce the reinfection risk.

Physiotherapist

PJI is a complex problem that requires a multidisciplinary and coordinated approach amongst clinicians and healthcare professionals. Patients undergoing revision surgery for PJI often have complex and unmet needs. Pre- and post-operative physiotherapy can lead to faster restoration of activity and function. It has been shown that patients undergoing revision surgery require enhanced support and integrated institutional pathways should be in place [61].

Nursing Specialists

An MDT meeting and care plan should also involve a dedicated nurse specialist in PJI. Their role in patient preparation, effective communication, inpatient care and support is of paramount importance through the surgical journey. They often coordinate care among several specialties, ensure the necessary tests and investigations are performed, provide organizational support, and act as a point of contact for patientswalker [62].

Many MDTs have begun with the participation of orthopedic specialists and microbiologists at first, and expand to involve more members, gradually increasing in size and complexity as the service evolves [44, 54]. Furthermore, the patient-specific medical needs should be considered, and relevant specialists should be invited on an ad hoc basis to pre-empt difficulties during the peri-operative period. Examples include, but not limited to, orthogeriatricians, diabetologists, and anesthesiologists.

Setting Up an MDT

The particular manner of organization of services varies from institution to institution and region, depending on the service array provided and the level of expertise available, the geographical make-up, the population, funding, and political organization of healthcare delivery at a national level.

Historically, most MDT meetings were likely to have involved most participants congregating in the same room. However, the COVID-19 pandemic has necessitated a major change in the MDT landscape. Applications like Zoom and Microsoft Teams have gained widespread popularity and are generally accepted to be secure and reliable [63]. Telemedicine MDT services have shown to be time effective, reduce overtime, build stable competence network, and increase expertise [64].

The hub-and spoke model design is a model which arranges service delivery into a network consisting of an anchor establishment (hub) which offers a full array of services, complemented by secondary establishments (spokes) which offer more limited-service arrays, routing patients needing more intensive and complex revisions to the hub for treatment. It is a much more efficient than organization designs which replicate operations across multiple sites. Hub-and-spoke networks are highly scalable, with satellites being added as needed or desired [65].

Following the "hub-and-spoke" model, the vast majority of revision arthroplasty is undertaken at the hub center. Revision procedures and emergency revisions cases are undertaken at satellite sites depending on the level of expertise, but all cases are discussed and reviewed at the regional MDT. Remote access through virtual platforms allows for all the centers to meet and discuss cases on a regular basis before any revision procedure is carried out.

There should be a standardized referral proforma and an MDT coordinator should promptly respond to all referrals and organizes for the images and cases to be presented at the MDT meeting. These proformas can be electronic or email based with specific word templates capturing all pertinent information including patient demographics, patient medical history, pertinent clinical information, and further investigations. Electronic referrals create an easily accessible audit trail and ensures all information is complete prior to the MDT. This will ensure that all patients are captured saved within the MDT work files and a central database, so their data is collected, captured, and not lost.

The MDT is not just a discussion forum, patients are referred into the service as part of a pathway. Some patients will be referred in purely for advice on antibiotics and the type of care agreed will be delivered locally, others will have their care transferred to the hub center for more specialist care throughout their journey. In complex cases when surgery is required, surgical planning is performed and details such as surgical approach, instruments, and required implants are all discussed. In addition, the MDT also reviews all post-operative revision arthroplasty imaging.

The MDT meetings typically last 1 h and it is important for the MDT outcome to be documented and uploaded online to the patients' archives to ensure accessibility to everyone involved in patient care. To that end, devising an MDT proforma with pre-specified outcomes and recommendations is key. Confirmation of the pre-operative plan and actual surgical intervention is reviewed and audited from the central database. This guarantees patient continuity of care and allows for integration of patient management and follow-up into research and audit purposes.

The MDT can further be augmented with integrated outpatient clinics. Carlson et al. [66] implemented a local clinical model, the arthroplasty infection service (AIS), to enhance coordination of care between their infectious disease clinicians and orthopedic arthroplasty surgeons for patient with PJI. This consisted of combined clinics, standardized lab testing, and planned revision procedures. Their model of combined clinics allowed their infectious disease to meet patients in a pre-operative clinic environment along with the orthopedic specialist. They infectious disease physicians appreciated the improved continuity of patient care and reduction in missed appointments [66].

There is evidence that better outcomes can be achieved by hospitals undertaking high volumes of particular specialist procedures [67]. Current principles recommend a multidisciplinary approach, along with a defined pathway, with new British Orthopaedic Association Standards for Trauma and Orthopaedics (BOAST) guidelines steering uniformity across units.

At a national level there is increasing appeal for delivery of complex PJI surgery at designated specialist centers. The French Health Ministry introduced a nationwide healthcare network with regional labeled centers in the management of bone and joint infections. The setting up of the CRIOAc (Centres de Référence des Infections Ostéoarticulaires complexes) network in France required considerable time and financial resources in which 24 dedicated centers were approved for treating bone and joint infections including PJI [68]. Over the course of 4 years, they saw a substantial rise in the incidence of case discussions and multidisciplinary meetings between orthopedists, ID physicians, and microbiologists. They concluded that the shared model enhanced PJI management, education, and research.

Personal and Team Skills Within an MDT

Good relationships between the teams and good communication with colleagues at various levels of hierarchy [38, 39], and managing disagreements within teams are recognized characteristics of an effective meeting chair, and is a key contribution to safe, high quality care delivery across specialities [37]. Good relationships between team members and adequate non-technical skills are important for smooth effective MDT functioning. Effective leadership of an MDT, which includes chairing of team meetings, can play an important role in ensuring equality and inclusiveness of participation that may enable better decision-making [41]. Disagreement should be seen as not detrimental to a team as it can enhance critical thinking and evaluation during decision-making, allow for open communication and differing techniques and methods to be discussed and avoid the risks of "group think" [69].

Having pathway coordinators with clear role descriptions allowing for collection of cases to be discussed, coordinate the dates and agenda for the meetings, document the discussions, and circulate the results of the meetings to all involved parties, members, and patients [70–72]. Some have standardized referral pathways and protocols (online resources or paper format referral pathways) for their units [54]. In a study by Goodson et al. [73], implementation of a fast-track PJI protocol managed by an orthopedic-specific infectious disease physician resulted in shorter hospital stays. Good record keeping of the discussion and agreed actions which are disseminated to all parties is a vital role of any MDT [74–76].

Support at an organizational level is also important, leadership at system or board level [77], and at operational level that will encourage attendance with protected time in the participants' job plans to prepare for, attend, and act on the workload of the meeting [78, 79].

The lack of protected time for team meetings are some barriers to effective meetings, with team members without protected time for meetings were less likely to attend [69], and that the most frequently cited organizational improvement to MDT working was more time dedicated to prepare for and attend the MDM [37]. Job planning for all the members of the team should be coordinated to allow all members to meet or dial in during their busy weekly schedule for the MDT to work.

Technology and decision support systems also play an important role. Telemedicine improves meeting attendance, allows for communication at a regional level and across several sites, and it is cost-effective. However, it can slow down the team by reducing the number of patient discussed per meeting [78] and can negatively affect the team's decision-making [80].

Conclusion

The treatment of PJI is labor and resource intensive. Patients often stay on the ward for extended periods and face a higher risk of surgical and medical complications that non-infected cases. Single-stage revision is an effective option for the infected TKA and, where appropriate, provides significant potential benefits for both for the patient and healthcare system. MDT meetings help synthesize the collective knowledge, experiences, and opinions from a range of specialists with the aim of streamlining the management of both acute and chronic medical conditions and disease processes. Its goal is to improve outcomes in a holistic bespoke manner. We advocate the role of a specialist infection MDT in the management of these patients to allow an individualized patient-centered approach and care plan and thereby reducing recurrence and reoperation rates.

References

1. Tande AJ, Patel R. Prosthetic joint infection. Clin Microbiol Rev. 2014;27(2):302–45. Epub 2014/04/04.
2. Chirca L, Marculescu C. Prevention of infection in orthopedic prosthetic surgery. Infect Dis Clin North Am. 2017;31(2):253.
3. Zimmerli W, Trampuz A, Ochsner PE. Current concepts: prosthetic-joint infections. N Engl J Med. 2004;351(16):1645–54.
4. NJR. NJR 18th annual report. In: Registry NJ, editor. National Joint Registry for England, Wales, Northern Ireland and the Isle of Man; 2021.
5. Blom AW, Brown J, Taylor AH, Pattison G, Whitehouse S, Bannister GC. Infection after total knee arthroplasty. J Bone Joint Surg Br. 2004;86(5):688–91. Epub 2004/07/28.
6. Patel A, Pavlou G, Mujica-Mota RE, Toms AD. The epidemiology of revision total knee and hip arthroplasty in England and Wales a comparative analysis with projections for the United States. A study using the national joint registry dataset. Bone Joint J. 2015;97B(8):1076–81.
7. Stone B, Nugent M, Young SW, Frampton C, Hooper GJ. The lifetime risk of revision following total knee arthroplasty : a New Zealand Joint Registry study. Bone Joint J. 2022;104-B(2):235–41. Epub 2022/02/01.
8. Kurtz S, Ong K, Lau E, Mowat F, Halpern M. Projections of primary and revision hip and knee arthroplasty in the United States from 2005 to 2030. J Bone Joint Surg Am Vol. 2007;89A(4):780–5.
9. Ahmed SS, Haddad FS. Prosthetic joint infection. Bone Joint Res. 2019;8(11):570–2.

10. Kallala RF, Vanhegan IS, Ibrahim MS, Sarmah S, Haddad FS. Financial analysis of revision knee surgery based on NHS tariffs and hospital costs: does it pay to provide a revision service? Bone Joint J. 2015;97B(2):197–201.
11. Zahar A, Kendoff DO, Klatte TO, Gehrke TA. Can good infection control be obtained in one-stage exchange of the infected TKA to a rotating hinge design? 10-year results. Clin Orthop Relat Res. 2016;474(1):81–7.
12. Macheras GA, Kateros K, Galanakos SP, Koutsostathis SD, Kontou E, Papadakis SA. The long-term results of a two-stage protocol for revision of an infected total knee replacement. J Bone Joint Surg Br. 2011;93B(11):1487–92.
13. Tibrewal S, Malagelada F, Jeyaseelan L, Posch F, Scott G. Single-stage revision for the infected total knee replacement: results from a single centre. Bone Joint J. 2014;96B(6):759–64.
14. Mortazavi SMJ, Vegari D, Ho A, Zmistowski B, Parvizi J. Two-stage exchange arthroplasty for infected total knee arthroplasty: predictors of failure. Clin Orthop Relat Res. 2011;469(11):3049–54.
15. Haddad FS, Sukeik M, Alazzawi S. Is single-stage revision according to a strict protocol effective in treatment of chronic knee arthroplasty infections? Clin Orthop Relat Res. 2015;473(1):8–14.
16. Kini SG, Gabr A, Das R, Sukeik M, Haddad FS. Two-stage revision for periprosthetic hip and knee joint infections. Open Orthop J. 2016;2016(10):579–88.
17. Gooding CR, Masri BA, Duncan CP, Greidanus NV, Garbuz DS. Durable infection control and function with the PROSTALAC spacer in two-stage revision for infected knee arthroplasty. Clin Orthop Relat Res. 2011;469(4):985–93.
18. Matar HE, Bloch BV, Snape SE, James PJ. Outcomes of single- and two-stage revision total knee arthroplasty for chronic periprosthetic joint infection: long-term outcomes of changing clinical practice in a specialist centre. Bone Joint J. 2021;103-b(8):1373–9. Epub 2021/08/03.
19. van den Kieboom J, Tirumala V, Box H, Oganesyan R, Klemt C, Kwon YM. One-stage revision is as effective as two-stage revision for chronic culture-negative periprosthetic joint infection after total hip and knee arthroplasty: a retrospective cohort study. Bone Joint J. 2021;103B(3):515–21.
20. Slullitel PA, Oñativia JI, Zanotti G, Comba F, Piccaluga F, Buttaro MA. One-stage exchange should be avoided in periprosthetic joint infection cases with massive femoral bone loss or with history of any failed revision to treat periprosthetic joint infection. Bone Joint J. 2021;103-b(7):1247–53. Epub 2021/07/02.
21. Oduwole KO, Molony DC, Walls RJ, Bashir SP, Mulhall KJ. Increasing financial burden of revision total knee arthroplasty. Knee Surg Sports Traumatol Arthrosc. 2010;18(7):945–8.
22. Iorio R, Healy WL, Richards JA. Comparison of the hospital cost of primary and revision total knee arthroplasty after cost containment. Orthopedics. 1999;22(2):195–9.
23. Wang CJ, Hsieh MC, Huang TW, Wang JW, Chen HS, Liu CY. Clinical outcome and patient satisfaction in aseptic and septic revision total knee arthroplasty. Knee. 2004;11(1):45–9.
24. Greidanus NV, Peterson RC, Masri BA, Garbuz DS. Quality of life outcomes in revision versus primary total knee arthroplasty. J Arthroplasty. 2011;26(4):615–20.
25. Barrack RL, Engh G, Rorabeck C, Sawhney J, Woolfrey M. Patient satisfaction and outcome after septic versus aseptic revision total knee arthroplasty. J Arthroplasty. 2000;15(8):990–3.
26. Baker JF, Stoyanov V, Shafqat A, Lui DF, Mulhall KJ. Total joint arthroplasty in nonagenarians—a retrospective review of complications and resource use. Acta Orthop Belg. 2012;78(6):745–50.
27. Klasan A, Schermuksnies A, Gerber F, Bowman M, Fuchs-Winkelmann S, Heyse TJ. Development of antibiotic resistance in periprosthetic joint infection after total knee arthroplasty. Bone Joint J. 2021;103-b(6 Suppl A):171–6. Epub 2021/06/01.
28. Marín M, Garcia-Lechuz JM, Alonso P, Villanueva M, Alcalá L, Gimeno M, et al. Role of universal 16S rRNA gene PCR and sequencing in diagnosis of prosthetic joint infection. J Clin Microbiol. 2012;50(3):583–9. Epub 2011/12/16.

29. Ji B, Li G, Zhang X, Xu B, Wang Y, Chen Y, et al. Effective single-stage revision using intra-articular antibiotic infusion after multiple failed surgery for periprosthetic joint infection: a mean seven years' follow-up. Bone Joint J. 2022;104-b(7):867–74. Epub 2022/07/02.
30. Neufeld ME, Liechti EF, Soto F, Linke P, Busch SM, Gehrke T, et al. High revision rates following repeat septic revision after failed one-stage exchange for periprosthetic joint infection in total knee arthroplasty. Bone Joint J. 2022;104B(3):386–93.
31. Yapp LZ, Clement ND, Moran M, Clarke JV, Simpson A, Scott CEH. Long-term mortality rates and associated risk factors following primary and revision knee arthroplasty: 107,121 patients from the Scottish Arthroplasty Project. Bone Joint J. 2022;104-b(1):45–52. Epub 2022/01/01.
32. Moyad TF, Thornhill T, Estok D. Evaluation and management of the infected total hip and knee. Orthopedics. 2008;31(6):581–8.
33. Ibrahim MS, Raja S, Khan MA, Haddad ES. A multidisciplinary team approach to two-stage revision for the infected hip replacement. Bone Joint J. 2014;96B(10):1312–8.
34. Rosell L, Alexandersson N, Hagberg O, Nilbert M. Benefits, barriers and opinions on multidisciplinary team meetings: a survey in Swedish cancer care. BMC Health Serv Res. 2018;18:249.
35. Ellis PM. The importance of multidisciplinary team management of patients with non-small-cell lung cancer. Curr Oncol. 2012;19:S7–S15.
36. Freeman RK, Van Woerkom JM, Vyverberg A, Ascioti AJ. The effect of a multidisciplinary thoracic malignancy conference on the treatment of patients with esophageal cancer. Ann Thorac Surg. 2011;92(4):1239–42.
37. Soukup T, Lamb BW, Arora S, Darzi A, Sevdalis N, Green JS. Successful strategies in implementing a multidisciplinary team working in the care of patients with cancer: an overview and synthesis of the available literature. J Multidiscip Healthc. 2018;11:49–61. Epub 2018/02/07.
38. Soukup T, Lamb BW, Sarkar S, Arora S, Shah S, Darzi A, et al. Predictors of treatment decisions in multidisciplinary oncology meetings: a quantitative observational study. Ann Surg Oncol. 2016;23(13):4410–7. Epub 2016/11/03.
39. Soukup T, Petrides KV, Lamb BW, Sarkar S, Arora S, Shah S, et al. The anatomy of clinical decision-making in multidisciplinary cancer meetings a cross-sectional observational study of teams in a natural context. Medicine. 2016;95(24):e3885.
40. Lamb B, Green JSA, Vincent C, Sevdalis N. Decision making in surgical oncology. Surg Oncol. 2011;20(3):163–8.
41. Lamb B, Payne H, Vincent C, Sevdalis N, Green JSA. The role of oncologists in multidisciplinary cancer teams in the UK: an untapped resource for team leadership? J Eval Clin Pract. 2011;17(6):1200–6.
42. Lamb BW, Jalil RT, Sevdalis N, Vincent C, Green JSA. Strategies to improve the efficiency and utility of multidisciplinary team meetings in urology cancer care: a survey study. BMC Health Serv Res. 2014;14:377.
43. Akgun D, Muller M, Perka C, Winkler T. High cure rate of periprosthetic hip joint infection with multidisciplinary team approach using standardized two-stage exchange. J Orthop Surg Res. 2019;14:78.
44. Biddle M, Kennedy JW, Wright PM, Ritchie ND, Meek RMD, Rooney BP. Improving outcomes in acute and chronic periprosthetic hip and knee joint infection with a multidisciplinary approach. Bone Jt Open. 2021;2(7):509–14.
45. Ntalos D, Berger-Groch J, Rohde H, Grossterlinden LG, Both A, Luebke A, et al. Implementation of a multidisciplinary infections conference affects the treatment plan in prosthetic joint infections of the hip: a retrospective study. Arch Orthop Trauma Surg. 2019;139(4):467–73.
46. Vuorinen M, Makinen T, Rantasalo M, Huotari K. Effect of a multidisciplinary team on the treatment of hip and knee prosthetic joint infections: a single-centre study of 154 infections. Infect Dis. 2021;53(9):700–6.
47. Razii N, Clutton JM, Kakar R, Morgan-Jones R. Single-stage revision for the infected total knee arthroplasty: the Cardiff experience. Bone Jt Open. 2021;2(5):305–13. Epub 2021/05/19.

48. Parvizi J, Zmistowski B, Berbari EF, Bauer TW, Springer BD, Della Valle CJ, et al. New definition for periprosthetic joint infection: from the workgroup of the musculoskeletal infection society. Clin Orthop Relat Res. 2011;469(11):2992–4.
49. Parvizi J, Jacovides C, Zmistowski B, Jung KA. Definition of periprosthetic joint infection: is there a consensus? Clin Orthop Relat Res. 2011;469(11):3022–30.
50. Oussedik S, Gould K, Stockley I, Haddad FS. Defining peri-prosthetic infection: do we have a workable gold standard? J Bone Joint Surg Br. 2012;94B(11):1455–6.
51. Diaz-Ledezma C, Higuera CA, Parvizi J. Success after treatment of periprosthetic join infection: a Delphi-based international multidisciplinary consensus. Clin Orthop Relat Res. 2013;471(7):2374–82.
52. Lamb BW, Brown KF, Nagpal K, Vincent C, Green JSA, Sevdalis N. Quality of care management decisions by multidisciplinary cancer teams: a systematic review. Ann Surg Oncol. 2011;18(8):2116–25.
53. Lamb BW, Green JS, Benn J, Brown KF, Vincent CA, Sevdalis N. Improving decision making in multidisciplinary tumor boards: prospective longitudinal evaluation of a multicomponent intervention for 1,421 patients. J Am Coll Surg. 2013;217(3):412–20. Epub 2013/07/31.
54. Awad F, Searle D, Walmsley K, Dyar N, Auckland C, Bethune R, et al. The exeter knee infection multi disciplinary team approach to managing prosthetic knee infections: a qualitative analysis. J Orthop. 2020;18:86–90. Epub 2020/03/20.
55. Jenkins N, Hughes H. How I do it…. How infection doctors approach the PJI MDT. Knee. 2020;27(6):1994–7. Epub 2020/11/18.
56. Li HK, Scarborough M, Zambellas R, Cooper C, Rombach I, Walker AS, et al. Oral versus intravenous antibiotic treatment for bone and joint infections (OVIVA): study protocol for a randomised controlled trial. Trials. 2015;16:583. Epub 2015/12/23.
57. Scarborough M, Li HK, Rombach I, Zambellas R, Walker AS, McNally M, et al. Oral versus intravenous antibiotics for bone and joint infections: the OVIVA non-inferiority RCT. Health Technol Assess. 2019;23(38):1–92. Epub 2019/08/03.
58. Li HK, Rombach I, Zambellas R, Walker AS, McNally MA, Atkins BL, et al. Oral versus intravenous antibiotics for bone and joint infection. N Engl J Med. 2019;380(5):425–36.
59. Yi PH, Frank RM, Vann E, Sonn KA, Moric M, Della Valle CJ. Is potential malnutrition associated with septic failure and acute infection after revision total joint arthroplasty? Clin Orthop Relat Res. 2015;473(1):175–82. Epub 2014/05/29.
60. Blevins K, Aalirezaie A, Shohat N, Parvizi J. Malnutrition and the development of periprosthetic joint infection in patients undergoing primary elective total joint arthroplasty. J Arthroplast. 2018;33(9):2971–5. Epub 2018/05/16.
61. Moore AJ, Whitehouse MR, Gooberman-Hill R, Heddington J, Beswick AD, Blom AW, et al. A UK national survey of care pathways and support offered to patients receiving revision surgery for prosthetic joint infection in the highest volume NHS Orthopaedic Centres. Musculoskeletal Care. 2017;15(4):379–85. Epub 2017/03/24.
62. Walker J. Care of patients undergoing joint replacement. Nurs Older People. 2012;24(1):14–20. Epub 2012/03/22.
63. Currie GP, Kennedy AM, Chetty M. COVID-19 and the multidisciplinary team meeting: 'should old acquaintance be forgot?'. J R Coll Physicians Edinb. 2021;51(4):327–9. Epub 2021/12/10.
64. Aghdam MRF, Vodovnik A, Hameed RA. Role of telemedicine in multidisciplinary team meetings. J Pathol Inform. 2019;10:35. Epub 2019/12/05.
65. Elrod JK, Fortenberry JL Jr. The hub-and-spoke organization design: an avenue for serving patients well. BMC Health Serv Res. 2017;17(Suppl 1):457. Epub 2017/07/20.
66. Carlson VR, Dekeyser GJ, Certain L, Pupaibool J, Gililland JM, Anderson LA. Clinical experience with a coordinated multidisciplinary approach to treating prosthetic joint infection. Arthroplast Today. 2020;6(3):360–2.
67. Katz JN, Losina E, Barrett J, Phillips CB, Mahomed NN, Lew RA, et al. Association between hospital and surgeon procedure volume and outcomes of total hip replacement in the United States Medicare population. J Bone Joint Surg Am. 2001;83A(11):1622–9.

68. Ferry T, Seng P, Mainard D, Jenny JY, Laurent F, Senneville E, et al. The CRIOAc healthcare network in France: a nationwide health ministry program to improve the management of bone and joint infection. Orthop Traumatol Surg Res. 2019;105(1):185–90. Epub 2018/11/11.
69. Lamb BW, Taylor C, Lamb JN, Strickland SL, Vincent C, Green JSA, et al. Facilitators and barriers to teamworking and patient centeredness in multidisciplinary cancer teams: findings of a national study. Ann Surg Oncol. 2013;20(5):1408–16.
70. Balfour A, Burch J, Fecher-Jones I, Carter FJ. Exploring the fundamental aspects of the enhanced recovery after surgery nurse's role. Nurs Stand. 2019;34:70. Epub 2019/11/12.
71. Palese A, Comuzzi C, Bresadola V. Global case management: the "nurse case manager" model applied to day surgery in Italy. Lippincotts Case Manag. 2005;10(2):83–92. Epub 2005/04/09.
72. Escobar MA, Brewer A, Caviglia H, Forsyth A, Jimenez-Yuste V, Laudenbach L, et al. Recommendations on multidisciplinary management of elective surgery in people with haemophilia. Haemophilia. 2018;24(5):693–702. Epub 2018/06/27.
73. Goodson KM, Kee JR, Edwards PK, Novack AJ, Stambough JB, Siegel ER, et al. Streamlining hospital treatment of prosthetic joint infection. J Arthroplast. 2020;35(3S):S63–S8. Epub 2020/02/13.
74. Palmer JE, Wales K, Ellis K, Dudding N, Smith J, Tidy JA. The multidisciplinary colposcopy meeting: recommendations for future service provision and an analysis of clinical decision making. BJOG. 2010;117(9):1060–6. Epub 2010/07/08.
75. Gandara E, Ungar J, Lee J, Chan-Macrae M, O'Malley T, Schnipper JL. Discharge documentation of patients discharged to subacute facilities: a three-year quality improvement process across an integrated health care system. Jt Comm J Qual Patient Saf. 2010;36(6):243–51. Epub 2010/06/23.
76. Drew S, Judge A, Cohen R, Fitzpatrick R, Barker K, Gooberman-Hill R. Enhanced recovery after surgery implementation in practice: an ethnographic study of services for hip and knee replacement. BMJ Open. 2019;9(3):e024431. Epub 2019/03/08.
77. Kemper-Koebrugge W, Koetsenruijter J, Rogers A, Laurant M, Wensing M. Local networks of community and healthcare organisations: a mixed methods study. BMC Res Notes. 2016;9:331. Epub 2016/07/03.
78. Lamb BW, Sevdalis N, Arora S, Pinto A, Vincent C, Green JSA. Teamwork and team decision-making at multidisciplinary cancer conferences: barriers, facilitators, and opportunities for improvement. World J Surg. 2011;35(9):1970–6.
79. Raine R, Wallace I, Nic a' Bháird C, Xanthopoulou P, Lanceley A, Clarke A, et al. Improving the effectiveness of multidisciplinary team meetings for patients with chronic diseases: a prospective observational study. Southampton: NIHR Journals Library; 2014. Copyright © Queen's Printer and Controller of HMSO 2014.
80. Jalil R, Lamb B, Russ S, Sevdalis N, Green JS. The cancer multi-disciplinary team from the coordinators' perspective: results from a national survey in the UK. BMC Health Serv Res. 2012;12:457. Epub 2012/12/15.

Surgical Technique, Bone Loss, and Muscle Insufficiency

Bernd Fink

Introduction

In recent years, it has been shown that the outcomes of one-stage septic prosthesis revisions of the knee joint are comparable in terms of freedom from infection and even slightly better in terms of clinical outcomes than two-stage revisions [1–5]. Panguard et al. [4], in a literature review of 14 articles with one-stage septic knee prosthesis revision in 687 patients, found an average infection-free rate of 87.1% compared with 84.8% in 1086 patients in 18 articles with two-stage septic knee prosthesis revision. The mean Knee Society score tended to be slightly better at 80.0 points for one-stage revision compared with 77.8 points for two-stage revision. Lenguerrand et al. [5] even observed a lower re-revision rate after one-stage revision than after two-stage knee prosthesis revision in their analysis of the National Joint Register for England and Wales (1.2 vs. 2.2, $p < 0.001$). Mortality 6 and 18 months after surgery was significantly lower after one-stage prosthesis revision than after two-stage revision (hazard ratio at 6 months 0.51, $p = 0.0049$; hazard ratio at 18 months 0.33, $p = 0.048$). Thus, it is clear that this concept is becoming more widely adopted for a certain cohort of patients.

One-stage septic knee prosthesis revision has the advantages of only one operation and the associated lower morbidity, shorter hospital stay and the associated lower cost, and better functional outcome. However, successful one-stage septic revision surgery requires patient selection and a specific surgical procedure. Thus, preoperative identification of the microorganism causing the infection is a basic requirement for one-stage revision surgery so that local and systemic specific antibiotic therapy can be selected based on the susceptibility of the microorganism. Polymicrobial infections and infections with atypical, gram-negative, or multidrug-resistant

---

B. Fink (✉)
Department of Joint Replacement and Revision Arthroplasty, Orthopaedic Clinic Markgröningen, Markgröningen, Germany
e-mail: bernd.fink@rkh-gesundheit.de

© The Author(s), under exclusive license to Springer Nature Switzerland AG 2024
M. Citak et al. (eds.), *One-Stage Septic Revision Arthroplasty*, https://doi.org/10.1007/978-3-031-59160-0_5

pathogens are not readily amenable to the alternative calculated antibiotic regimens otherwise used, so higher failure rates have been described for such cases [3, 6]. Although the ENDO-Klinik Hamburg also reported good outcomes of one-stage revision surgery with resistant microorganisms (with an infection-free rate of 93% after 10 years in all one-stage knee prosthesis revisions) [7], the following indications and relative contraindications for one-stage septic knee prosthesis revision have been defined at the International Consensus Meeting in 2018 [8]:

Indications for One-Stage Septic Exchange of the Knee

- PJI after TKA in which infection is proven based on the International Consensus Group on Periprosthetic Infection of PJI (at least one major or three minor criteria of at least 6 points according to the new definition) [8].
- Late or chronic infection more than 30 days postoperatively or hematogenous infection more than 30 days after onset of the symptoms.
- Known germ with known susceptibility based on microbiological diagnostics.
- Proper bone stock for fixation of cemented implants or uncemented reconstruction.
- Possibility of local and systemic antibiotic therapy.
- Possibility of primary wound closure (adequate condition of soft tissues).

Contraindications of One-Stage Procedure

- Culture-negative PJI.
- Lack of appropriate antibiotics.
- Systemic sepsis of the patient.
- Failure of two or more previous one-stage procedures [9].
- Infection involving the neurovascular bundles.
- Extensive soft tissue involvement that would prevent closure of the wound (Fig. 1).
- Infection with a highly virulent organism (difficult to treat microorganism), especially cases for which appropriate antibiotic-impregnated cement is not available.

Surgical Technique

During the revision surgery, removal of all foreign material (implant, cement) and extensive debridement is mandatory as the first steps and free bleeding in the periarticular soft tissue and bone should be achieved. All membranes (especially for the posterior capsule) and all well-fixed cement particles must be removed. During debridement, all necrotic bone has to be removed, all areas of osteolysis must be cleaned and a complete synovectomy has to be performed. Numerous samples must be taken for microbiologic evaluation from all periarticular areas, especially from the femoral and tibial intramedullary canals and the synovia. Special extraction instruments may be needed for the removal of the implants and have to be ordered for the particular implant in advance. Therefore, the identification of the

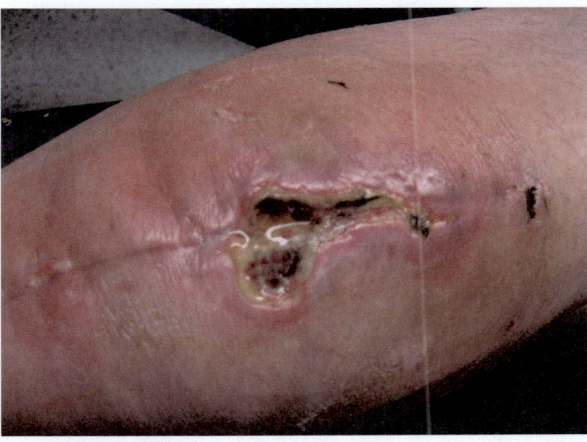

Fig. 1 Late periprosthetic infection of the knee joint with soft tissue damage precluding one-stage revision because of the impossibility of primary wound closure

type and manufacturer of the endoprosthesis is mandatory during preoperative planning.

Surface replacement prostheses (bicondylar prostheses) and infected unicompartmental prostheses can be released from their fixation by sawing underneath with a thin oscillating saw blade, a jigsaw or, if necessary, a Gigli saw, as well as by additional chiseling underneath (Fig. 2a–d). Removal of fixed stemmed prostheses is considerably more difficult. First, again, sawing and, if necessary, chiseling is performed below the articular surfaces of the prosthetic components. In the case of monoblock components with a tapered cemented stem, the components can usually be easily knocked out of the prosthesis bed. This is much more difficult for cylindrical stems. If these are attached to the articular surface components in a modular fashion, after the initial undercutting and chiseling, the stem should be disconnected from the surface component by disengaging the connection linkage and the surface component removed. Now the stem can be accessed, and can be chiseled around or, if necessary, reamed with a hollow reamer. Cementless, firmly seated stems can be loosened with thin flexible special chisels (e.g., Osteoclast flexible pneumatic chisel, Endocon, Neckargemünd, Germany). After loosening the stem, the upper component can then be reattached to the stem and the implant driven out by hitting the upper component. If this is not successful (e.g., in the case of very firmly attached cementless stems with a roughened surface) (Fig. 3), bone windows may have to be created in order to loosen the stems by chiseling and sawing around them. A tibial tubercle osteotomy is suitable for this purpose. Care must be taken later to close this window correctly so that cement cannot penetrate the osteotomy surfaces during one-stage implantation of the new prosthesis and thus prevent healing of the bony flap. Segur et al. [10] performed tubercle osteotomy in 26 cases of knee prosthesis revision following setting of a static spacer between the first and second stages of surgery and reported tubercle healing without complications 22 times (84.6%) and freedom from infection in 23 cases (88.4%) after an average of 3.4 years.

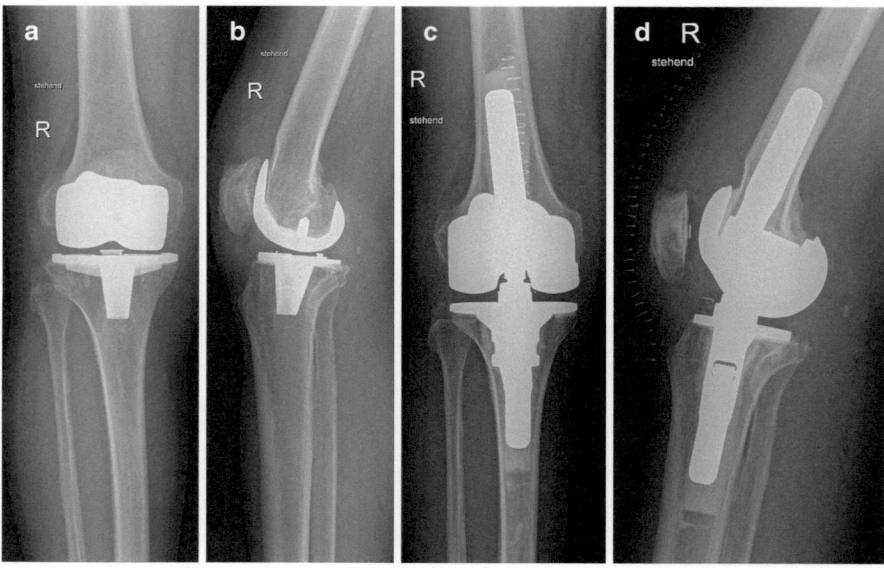

Fig. 2 Late infection of a surface replacement arthroplasty (**a**, **b**) with one-stage revision to an axis-guided prosthesis (**c**, **d**)

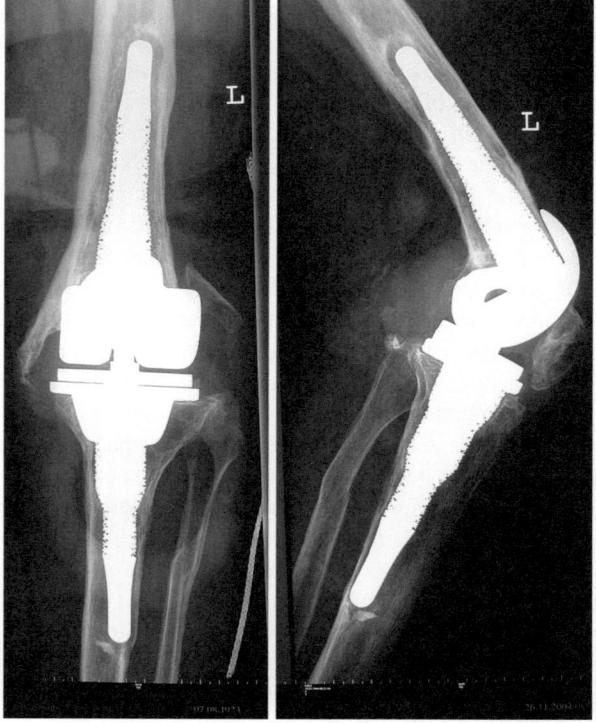

Fig. 3 Late infection of a cementless axis-guided knee endoprosthesis with rough surface structure

After removal of the cemented implants, the remaining cement must be removed. In the case of articular surface prostheses undergoing revision, this can be removed relatively easily using various chisels from the femoral condyles and the tibial plateau as well as, if necessary, from the metaphysis of the tibia. Removal from the diaphysis of the femur and tibia becomes more difficult with cemented stem prostheses. A large assortment of different chisels with different bevels and cutting directions is just as helpful as an assortment of long ball gouges, drills, sharp curettes, and taps. A number of special instruments has been developed for removal of the cement that can also be helpful. For example, the OSCAR system (Endocon, Neckargemünd, Germany) uses ultrasound technology for bone cement removal: the oscillating instrument tip emits ultrasonic waves that soften the cement locally and enable it to be scraped away.

Step-by-step ball reaming has proven effective for cement removal, initially to thin out the firmly adherent cement mantle. The thinner cement layer can then be removed in stages. Thinning the cement mantle in that first step reduces the risk of unintentional periprosthetic fractures during chiseling. The cement mantle is split longitudinally and radially using a sharp chisel with a tip ground on both sides (e.g., a nose chisel) and the individual cement pieces are then detached from the bone in pieces using a chisel ground on only one side. The individual pieces are separated from the bone by tilting the chisel into the femur/tibia or rotating the chisel. Swiveling the chisel against the bone is not recommended because of the risk of fractures.

More difficult is the removal of the distal, diaphyseal cement mantle, which is usually even more firmly seated than the proximal, metaphyseal one. There are a number of techniques with different functionalities, the use of which depends on the stability of the distal cement mantle. For example, the distal cement mantle can be drilled out stepwise. An intramedullary guide may be used for drilling to ensure that the drill is centered. A tap is then screwed into this drill hole. The thickest possible tap that can be screwed in is always used. Hammer blows against the head of the tap can then remove the attached cement ring. The tap should not be screwed in too deeply. Removing smaller cement pieces step by step is better and less risky than trying to remove a large, firmly seated cement piece, which would require considerably more force. This method only works with an intact cement mantle. If the cement mantle is incomplete at any point, the tap could be pushed against the softer bone and may damage it during further proceedings.

An easily accessible, short distal piece of cement can be drilled through completely and the hole can be enlarged slowly with thicker and thicker drills. In this case, we start with a long 4.5 mm drill, followed by 6 and 8 mm diameter drills. A retrograde chisel can then be passed through this hole, which then allows cement pieces to be knocked out in a retrograde direction.

Another method is to remove the distal cement mantle using the OSCAR system. The distal cement mantle is gradually softened by ultrasound and can then be scraped off in a series of gradual steps. Alternatively, the cement is softened and broken up into spaghetti-like strips, which are then allowed to harden again around the ultrasonic probe and be driven out with the probe using a slotted hammer.

Once the cement has been removed, it is important to check that the femur has not been perforated. A sensor can be inserted into the femur for this purpose and the inner wall scanned. Examination with a fluoroscope can also be helpful for this purpose.

Perforations and fractures should be bridged with the stem during the subsequent implantation of the new prosthetic component, thus influencing the choice of stem length.

After removal of all foreign material and radical debridement of the bone and soft tissues, irrigation with antiseptic solutions is useful for treating the wound bed [1, 11]. Here, various solutions are offered and described in various publications; e.g., Octenisept (Schülke & Mayr GmbH, Norderstedt, Germany), Lavasept (BBraun, Melsungen, Germany), Povidone iodine, Chlorhexidine [1, 3, 11]. Octenisept has the advantage that it has a shorter exposure time of 3 min compared to, for example, 12 min for Lavasept. However, because it is toxic to tissues, its use requires extensive rinsing before the new prosthesis is implanted.

After local wound cleansing, changing gloves, drapes, light handles, and surgical instruments is recommended before implanting a new prosthesis [12, 13]. The type of new prosthesis depends, on the one hand, on the bone defects existing after debridement and, above all, on existing ligamentous instability. Since ligamentous instability of the joint and bony defects do usually occur after radical debridement, semiconstrained or constrained (rotating hinges) can be considered almost exclusively as prosthesis models (Fig. 2a–d). An exception may be the treatment of a periprosthetic infection of a unicondylar prosthesis. In one study, we were able to demonstrate an infection-free rate of 100% for one-stage revisions of infected unicondylar prostheses to surface replacement prostheses with medial tibial augmentation and tibial stem extension, as well as the best clinical outcomes with a Knee Society Score of 84.5 ± 14.66 points at 2 years compared with revisions to axis-guided prostheses (Figs. 4a, b and 5a, b) [1].

When re-implanting the new prosthesis, it is essential for its function that the joint line is taken into account and restored. For this purpose, the epicondyles of the femur and the fibula tip serve as reference points (if still present) [14]. Mostly, 2 cm

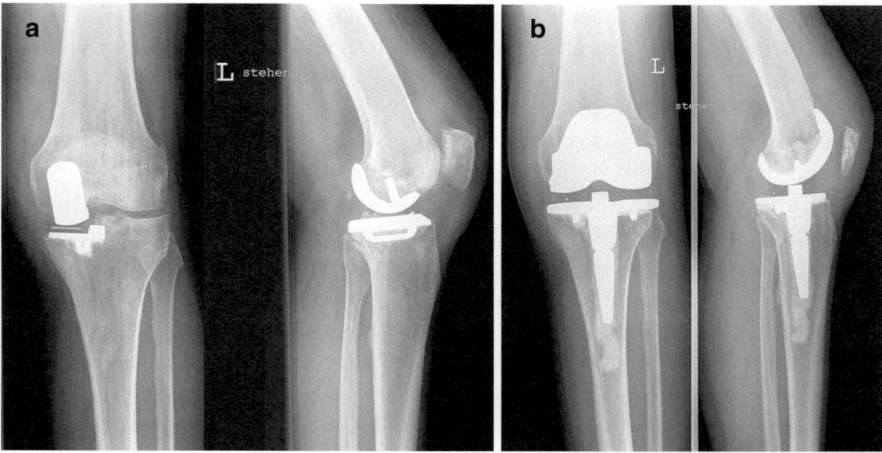

Fig. 4 Late infection of a unicondylar sled endoprosthesis (**a**) with one-stage revision to a surface replacement endoprosthesis with stem extension and filling of small cavitary defects with cement (**b**)

Surgical Technique, Bone Loss, and Muscle Insufficiency

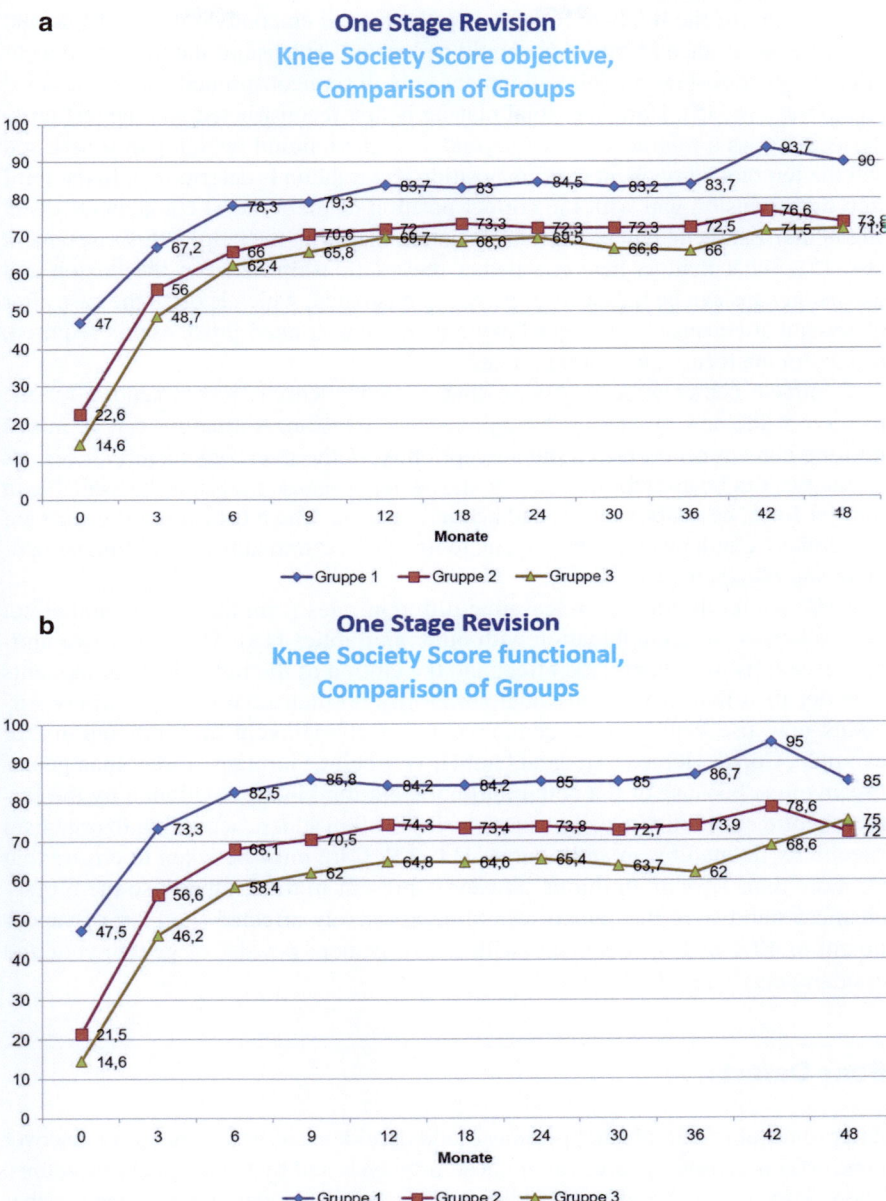

Fig. 5 Progression of Knee Society score (**a**) and functional Knee Society score (**b**) of one-stage revisions from 6 unicondylar sled prostheses to a surface replacement (blue line), 37 one-stage septic revisions from surface replacement prostheses to axis-guided prostheses (red line), and 20 axis-guided prostheses to axis-guided prostheses (green line)

above the tip of the fibula or 3 cm below the medial epicondyle the joint line and therefore the surface of the inlay should be located. The use of the three-step technique helps to restore the joint alignment in both semiconstrained and constrained prostheses [14, 15]. Here, the tibial plateau is first reconstructed and the test prosthesis is left as a reference. In the second step, the femoral flexion gap is assessed and the femoral component size, its position and rotation is determined. In the third step the extension gap with the correct position of the femoral component (distal augments) and the height of the inlay is determined with the help of this assessment [14, 15]. What matters here is whether the relationship between the flexion and extension gaps can be balanced. If there is a mismatch, which is often the case after debridement because of a larger flexion gap, a constrained prosthesis is required, usually in the form of a rotating hinge.

Complete cementation of the prosthesis components is recommended for the fixation of the new prosthesis during one-stage revision. Antibiotics can be mixed into the cement according to the susceptibility of the microorganism [7]. Not all antibiotics can be used for mixing into the cement because they must be available in powder form, be water-soluble, and be thermostable. The most commonly used are gentamicin, clindamycin, vancomycin, tobramycin, aztreonam, ampicillin, meropenem, and ofloxacin [16, 17].

Different antibiotics are released at different rates from the cement and affect each other when in combination with other antibiotics [18]. The use of two antibiotics results in a synergistic effect and the elution of the individual components is better than that of the individual antibiotics on their own [19–23]. Many surgeons now use cement with gentamycin and clindamycin in combination (for example, Copal, Heraeus Medical GmbH, Wertheim, Germany) rather than gentamycin alone because of the better antibiotic elution kinetics exhibited by the former; a third antibiotic (usually vancomycin) is often added, according to organism specificity defined by an antibiogram [11, 22]. Care must be taken to ensure that no more than 10% of antibiotic powder is present in total, otherwise the biomechanical stability of the cement would be negatively affected (i.e., 2 g of vancomycin in 40 g of Copal cement (with 2 g of cement powder of gentamycin and clindamycin)) [18, 19, 24].

Bone Defects

After removal of the infected prosthesis and debridement, it is common to discover bone defects caused by infection-induced osteolysis and by the surgical procedures. These defects must therefore be addressed during reimplantation of the new prosthesis. In principle, cement, morselized or structural allografts and metallic augments, cones or sleeves, and even megaprostheses can be used to build up the bone defects.

The disadvantage of using allografts in septic one-stage revision is firstly the risk of infection because they are non-vascularized osseous segments and may represent a potential sequestrum for microorganisms [25, 26]. Although there are individual reports of antibiotic-impregnated allografts being used in one-stage septic prosthesis revisions [27], the small number of cases means there is not enough data to unequivocally recommend their use in single septic prosthesis revisions.

The use of a classification for bone defects is helpful for managing bone defect strategy. Bone defects can be assessed in the preoperative radiographs and CT scans However, the extent of bone defects is not infrequently increased after intraoperative removal of implants and cement. The AORI (Anderson Orthopaedic Research Institute) has become generally accepted as the classification of bone defects [28–30]. Three types of defects are classified for the femur (F1, F2, F3) and tibia (T1, T2, T3), respectively. Each type is divided into "A" when one femoral condyle or one half of the tibial plateau is involved and "B" when both condyles and both halves of the tibial plateau are involved.

Type 1 defects include those with intact cortical bone and minor metaphyseal bone defects. These bone defects do not jeopardize the stability of the revision prosthetic component. In type 2 defects, there is a segmental defect with loss of cortical bone and damage to the metaphyseal bone that needs to be filled in with augments to restore the joint line. In type 3, the metaphyseal bone is significantly deficient. There is a severe bone loss affecting a significant portion of a femoral condyle up to the epicondyles or one of the tibial plateaus, producing knee instability due to injury of the corresponding collateral ligaments [31].

Bone cement with the added antibiotics is the best surgical option for filling bone defects of less than 5 mm in width and depth, in peripheral deficiencies of up to 10% of the femoral condylar area, in small central defects, in cystic defects, and in contained bone defects (Fig. 4b) [32]. Cement in combination with screws can be used for contained or uncontained defects measuring 5–10 mm in type 1 and type 2A defects, both in the distal femur and proximal tibia.

Augments (made of metal or PMMA) are used for uncontained defects. They serve to restore the joint line and to balance the soft tissue of the joint with regard to the flexion and extension gap [33]. During surgery, the bony articular surface is prepared with appropriate jigs and trial augments are placed on the trial prostheses on the surfaces near the joint under the tibial plateau and/or on the distal and posterior femoral articular surfaces of the femoral component. This can then be used to check whether the joint line has been set correctly and soft tissue balancing has been achieved (Figs. 6 and 8). It is also important to achieve these goals with the coupled prostheses as, otherwise, a non-physiologically high load would be placed on the axis of the prosthesis, which could cause failure of the implant over time [15].

Cones such as so-called trabecular metal cones or, more recently, titanium cones serve to provide metaphyseal support for the new prosthesis in the case of large cavitary or segmental defects of the metaphysis and also large cavitary defects at the meta-diaphyseal transition. In the latter case, the cavitary defects extend into the diaphysis. In this case, two cones can often be inserted one after the other to help provide support and fixation of the stemmed prosthesis close to the joint (Fig. 7a–e) [34]. Without this support, prostheses with long stems fixed solely with cementation would oscillate close to the joint, which would lead to early loosening of the prosthesis. This is also because of the significantly reduced interdigitation of the cement

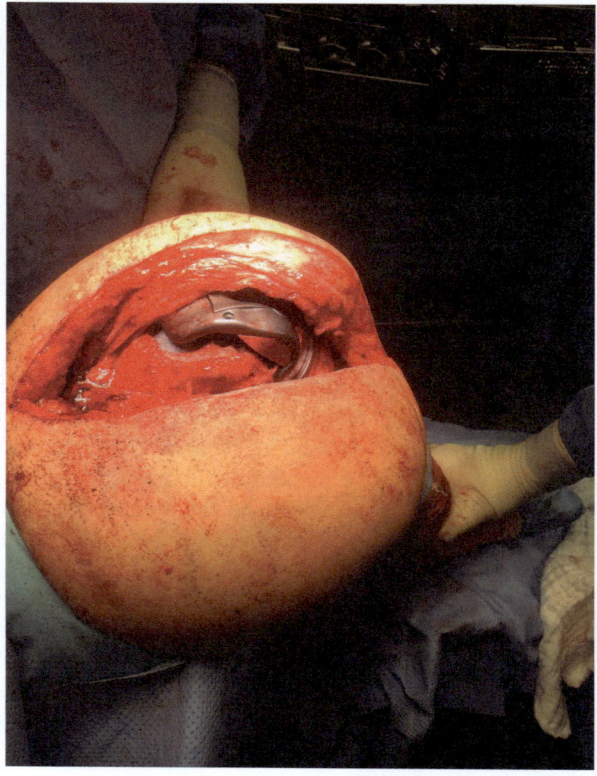

Fig. 6 Trial fitting of the prosthesis to assess the correct adjustment of the joint line

in the remaining, smooth bone surfaces with the resulting significantly reduced shear force stress at the bone cement interface. The contact surfaces of the cones are prepared in the bone with high-speed burs and shaping rasps and checked with trial cones. The trial components of the prosthesis are then inserted through the implanted trial cones with additional augments, if necessary, to check whether the prosthetic component can be implanted correctly (Fig. 8). The selected original cones are then carefully driven into place, undergoing press-fit fixation in the bone by means of their high surface roughness, their elasticity and the high level of friction involved. Interstices between the cones and the host bone can then be filled with allograft bone chips, whereby, for one-stage septic revision, these should be impregnated with an antibiotic powder (e.g., vancomycin). The prosthesis preassembled on the operating table with appropriate stem and augments is then cemented in place through the implanted cones (with specific antibiotic added to the cement). Burastero et al. [35] reported on 94 tantalum cones in 60 patients with two-stage septic knee prosthesis revision to constrained and semiconstrained knee prostheses with a mean follow-up of 43.5 ± 17.4 months. Two reinfections (3.3%) were observed, but no mechanical failure of the cones. The Knee Society Score and Oxford Knee Score

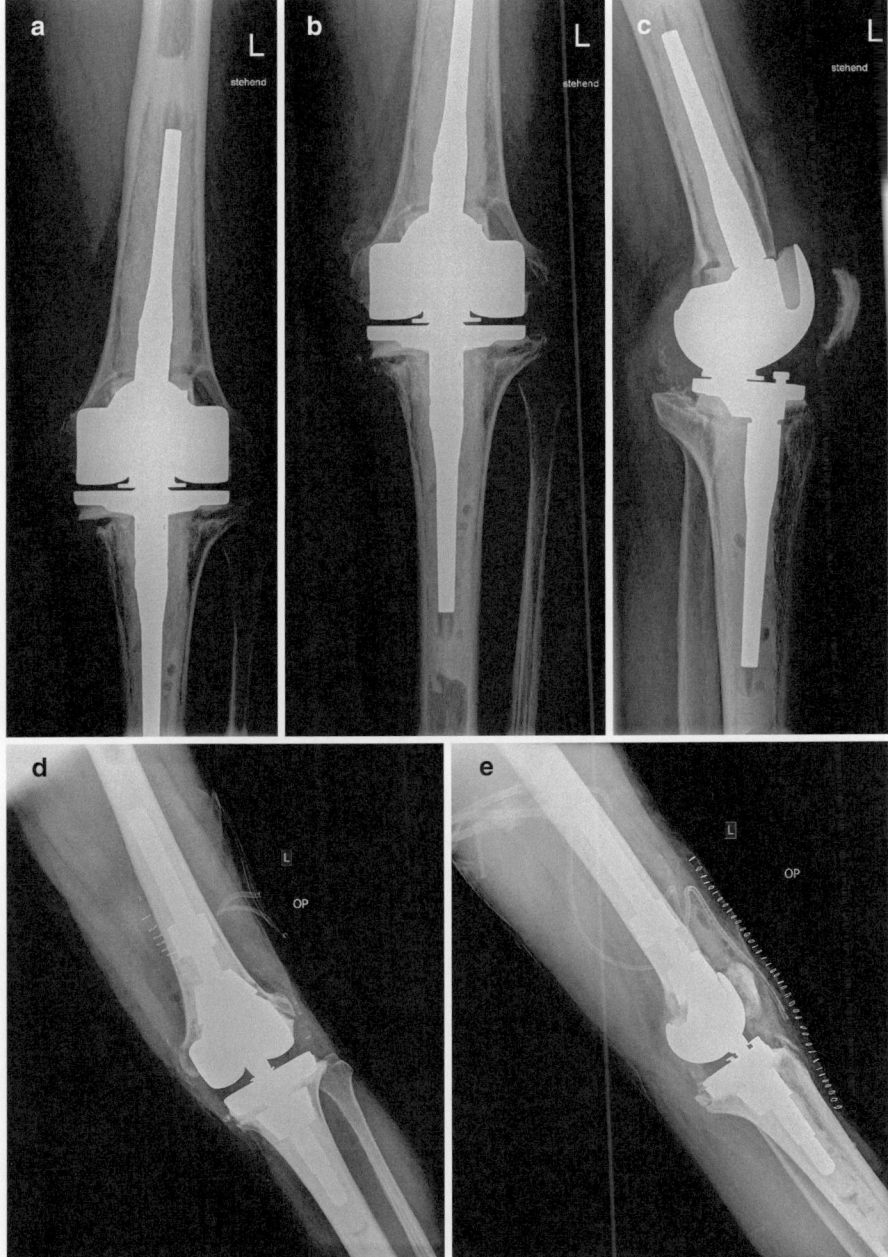

Fig. 7 One-stage septic revision of an axis-guided knee prosthesis (**a–c**) to an axis-guided knee prosthesis using two femoral cones and one tibial cone (**d, e**)

Fig. 8 Trial implantation of the trial prosthesis through the implanted femoral cone with distal augments

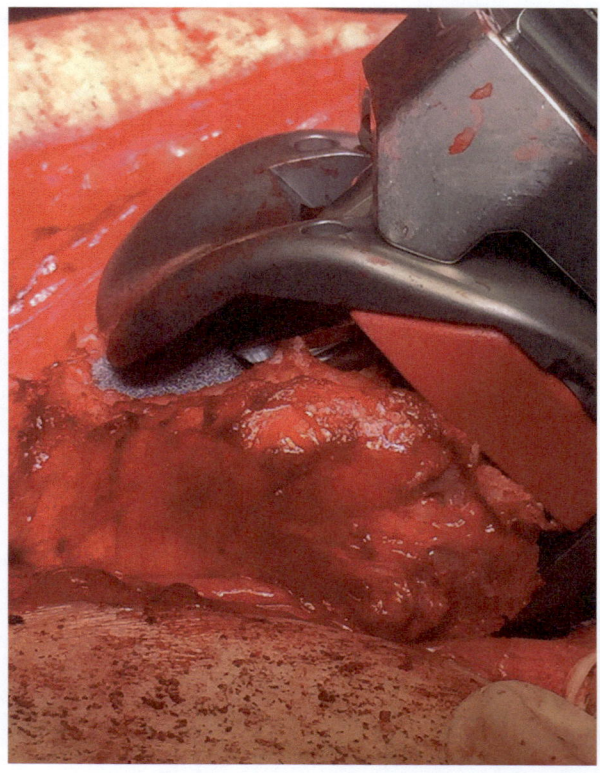

increased from 44.1 ± 7.4 points to 85.4 ± 5.6 points and from 19.2 ± 4.1 points to 38.4 ± 3.9 points, respectively. When indicated, we also use these cones in one-stage septic knee prosthesis revision because the reinfection rates are comparable to the two-stage procedure (Fig. 9a–d) [4, 5]. However, in cases of reinfection, removal of an osteointegrated cone is challenging. In this case, careful chiseling is required after prior stepwise removal of the cemented prosthesis (as described above).

Another method of management of bone defects is represented by sleeves, which are designed to effect better contact with the remaining healthy bone. They are suitable for large metaphyseal cavitary defects and are fixed to the implants and then implanted with them. Therefore, proper preparation of the host metaphyseal bone with appropriate shaping reamers or broaches is required to optimize the sleeve-bone contact. Klim et al. [36] studied 58 patients with a two-stage septic knee prosthesis replacement with sleeves an average of 5.3 years after surgery. They observed reinfection in 9 patients (16%) and American Knee Society score of 70 ± 20 points. The disadvantage of sleeves is that if reinfection occurs, they cannot be removed separately from the prosthesis, only the entire composite implant. In the case of a firmly fixed prosthesis, this requires a considerable amount of force with a corresponding risk of complications through periprosthetic fractures.

Surgical Technique, Bone Loss, and Muscle Insufficiency

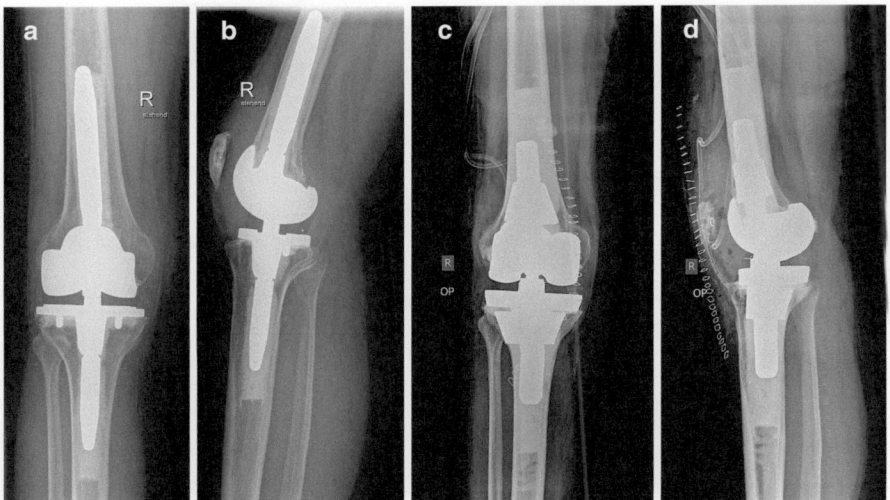

Fig. 9 One-stage septic revision of a semiconstrained knee prosthesis (**a, b**) to an axis-guided knee prosthesis using a femoral cone and a tibial cone (**c, d**)

In the case of pronounced segmental defects of the type AORI F3B or/and T3B, the only option is to use megaprostheses as distal femoral or/and proximal tibial replacements (Fig. 10a–d). This type of endoprosthetic owes its origins to the field of oncology where they are used for joint and limb preservation. Modular prosthetic components can be used to replace distal femoral or proximal tibial segments of different lengths and with the help of cementable stems they can be firmly fixed into the rest of the femur or tibia. If the defect extends far into the distal tibia and the attachment of the patellar tendon is also involved, as much healthy bone of the tibial tubercle as possible, with its patellar tendon attachment, should be fixed to the proximal tibial prosthesis [37]. The problem with megaprostheses is the large metal surface area, which is at high risk of bacterial colonization. For example, Smith et al. [38] found reinfection of 14 megaprostheses in 43% (6 cases) in septic two-stage revision surgery of the knee and Berend et al. [39] in 18% (2 of 11 patients).

Thus, the following recommendations can be made for reconstruction of bone defects during one-stage septic prosthesis revision:

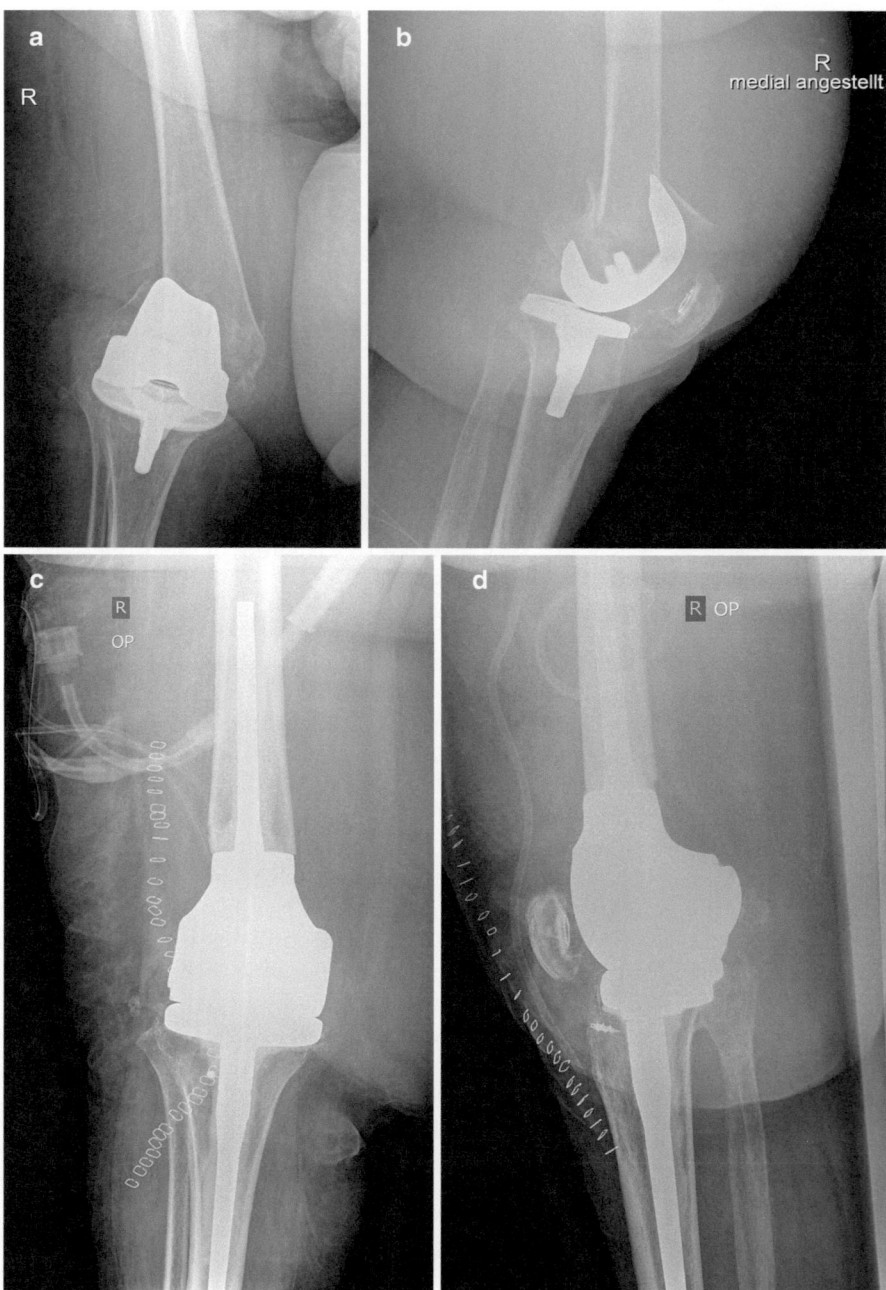

Fig. 10 One-stage septic revision of a surface prosthesis with periprosthetic fracture of the Rorabeck 3 type (**a, b**) to a distal femoral prosthesis (**c, d**)

AORI Type 1 Defects

Filling with cement alone is possible for contained bone defects less than 5 mm in diameter and depth (Figs. 2c, d and 4a, b). If the defects are larger, up to 1 cm in diameter and depth, the additional insertion of a screw is recommended, the head of which provides further support for the corresponding articular surface of the prosthetic component [40].

AORI Type 2 Defects

Small uncontained defects, again up to 5 mm in diameter and depth, can be filled with cement alone. Larger uncontained defects up to 1 cm in size and involving less than 50% of a femoral condyle or tibial plateau half, again require an additional stabilizing screw. Alternatively, augments can be used here as is the case for larger defects. However, the use of augments always requires a stemmed prosthesis (Fig. 7a–e) [32]. For even larger defects that cannot be filled with augments, the use of cones or sleeves is recommended (Fig. 9a–d).

AORI Type 3 Defects

For these large defects, only cones, sleeves, or megaprostheses can be considered. However, cones and sleeves still require sufficient press-fit fixation or support in the rest of the bone. If this no longer exists, only megaprostheses can be considered (Fig. 10a–d) [32].

Distal Femur Anatomy

Recently, a novel radiological classification system of the distal femur have been introduced (Fig. 11). According to the so-called Citak classification system [41], distal femur anatomy plays an important role for aseptic loosening following aseptic and septic revision surgery including the one-stage septic knee revision using rotating or full hinge knee prosthesis [42–45]. In a study by Scholz et al. [46], the aseptic loosening group following the one-stage septic exchange using hinge prostheses showed a high distribution of the Type C according to the Citak classification with 75.7% (Fig. 12). In this study, Type C femura had a sevenfold higher risk for aseptic loosening (AL). The distal femur anatomy is an independent risk factors for AL and should be determined preoperatively using plain radiographs. In patients with a wider canal of the femur or tibia, a cone or sleeve should be used to reduce the risk of AL.

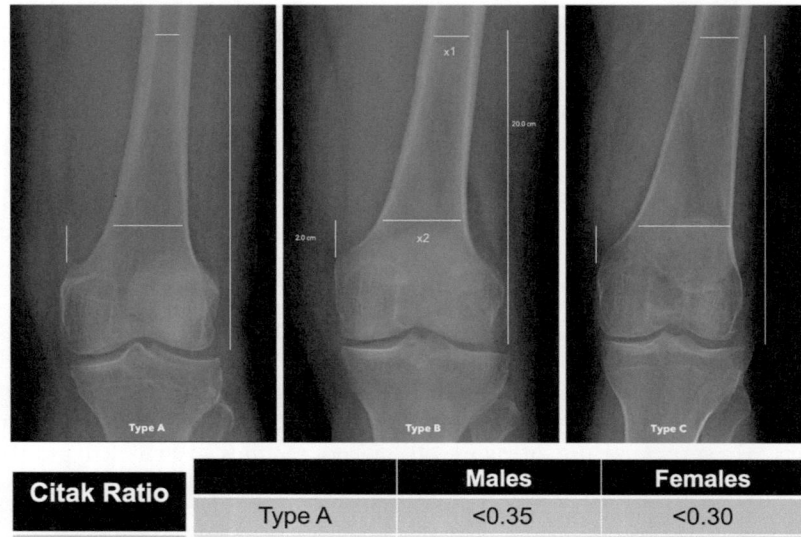

Fig. 11 Citak radiological classification system of the distal femur

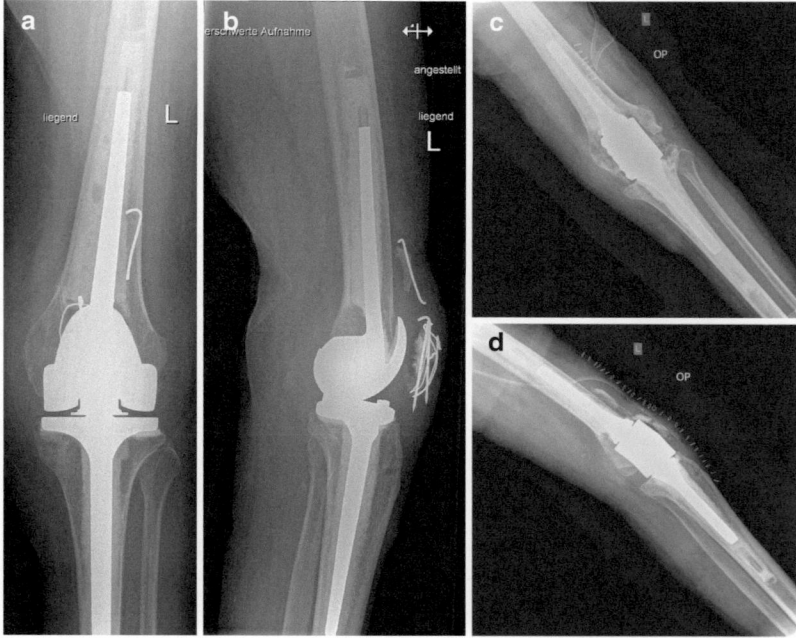

Fig. 12 One-stage septic revision of an axis-guided prosthesis with failed osteosynthesis of a patellar fracture and non-reconstructible extensor apparatus (**a, b**) to an arthrodesis rod (**c, d**)

Muscle Insufficiency

Muscle deficiencies in septic knee prosthesis revisions usually involve the extensor apparatus. This may be partly due to the need to remove the patellar component during a septic prosthesis revision. It is not mandatory to reimplant a resurfaced patella. Buller et al. [47] in a study of two-stage septic knee prosthesis revisions could not detect a significant difference, with regard to PROMs, between 43 patients with a resurfaced patellar component and 60 patients without. The remaining residual bone may also be insufficient for cementing in a new implant. However, if this would lead to an expected significant reduction in the strength of the extensor apparatus, suturing a trabecular metal patella into the thinned residual bone is recommended [48, 49].

If there is insufficiency of the quadriceps or patellar tendon because of, for example, infection and the need for debridement, these can be augmented with an autograft from below for the quadriceps tendon and from above for the patellar tendon [50–52]. If proximal tibial replacement is necessary, the goal should be to fix the patellar tendon to the proximal tibial graft with the still sufficient bony parts of the tubercle [37]. Sometimes artificial bands can support this fixation.

If reconstruction of the extensor apparatus is no longer possible, the only option is arthrodesis of the joint. In the case of periprosthetic infections, intramedullary arthrodesis rods cemented with an antibiotic specific for the bacterium causing the infection are recommended (Fig. 12a–d). While this can provide patients with pain relief, patient satisfaction with regard to functional outcome is low with this salvage procedure [53, 54]. Cones can also be used to securely support the arthrodesis rods in cases of concurrent bone defects (Fig. 13a–f).

If larger soft tissue defects exist that involve the extensor apparatus and do not allow primary wound closure, a muscle flap (usually gastrocnemius flap) can be used to cover them. To date such soft tissue defects have been discussed as a contraindication to one-stage septic knee prosthesis revision [8, 55, 56].

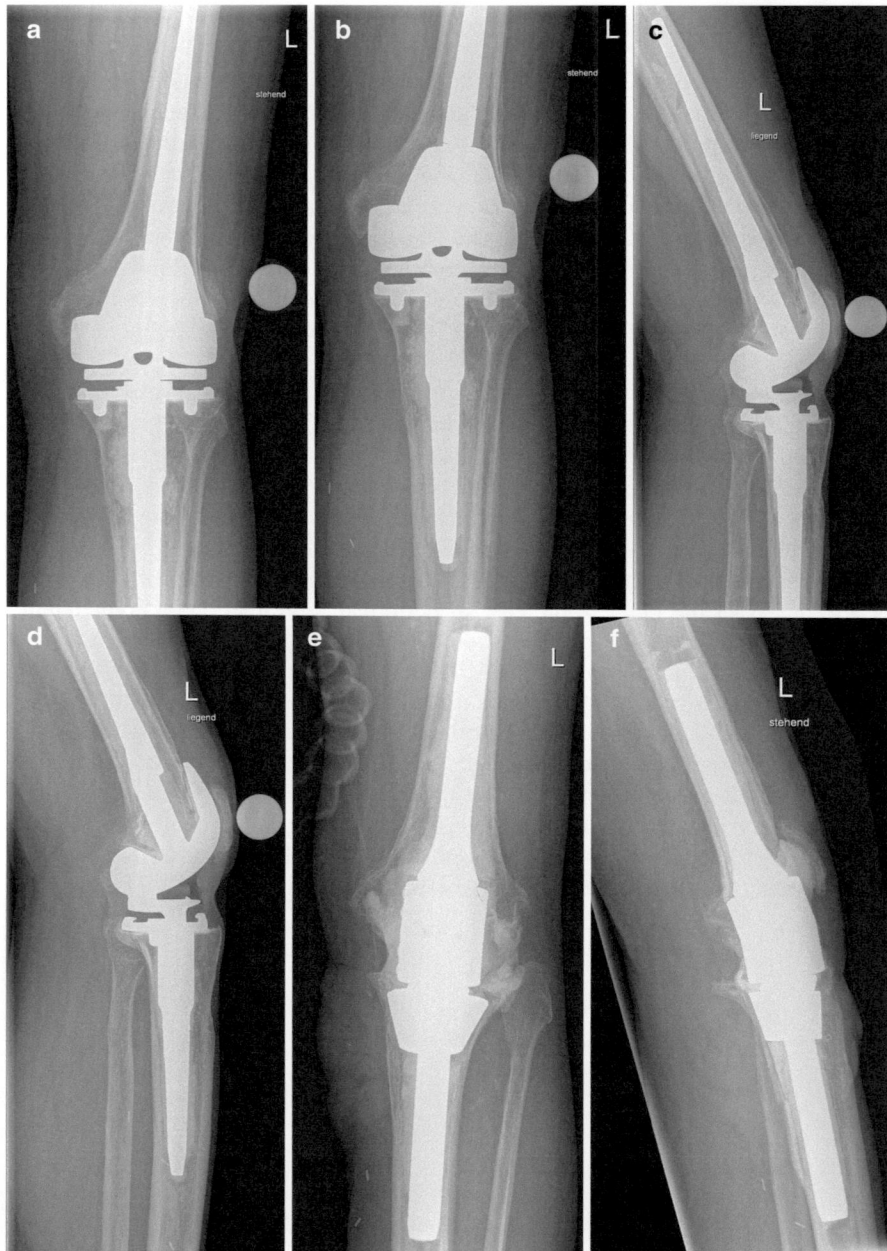

Fig. 13 One-stage septic revision of an axis-guided prosthesis with non-reconstructible extensor apparatus (**a–d**) to an arthrodesis rod with tibial cone (**e, f**)

References

1. Singer J, Merz A, Frommelt L, Fink B. High rate of infection control with one-stage revision of septic knee prostheses excluding MRSA and MRSE. Clin Orthop Relat Res. 2012;470:1461–71.
2. Lum ZC, Holland CT, Meehan JP. Systemic review of single stage revision for prosthetic joint infection. World J Orthop. 2020;11:559–72.
3. Tözün IR, Ozden VE, Dikmen G, Karaytug K. Trends in the treatment of infected knee arthro plasty. EFORT Open Rev. 2020;5:672–83.
4. Panguad C, Ollivier M, Argenson JN. Outcome of single-stage versus two-stage exchange for revision knee arthroplasty for chronic periprosthetic infection. EFFORT Open Rev. 2019;4:495–502.
5. Lenguerrand E, Whitehouse MR, Kunutsor SK, Beswick AD, Baker RP, Rolfson O, Reed MR, Blom AW. Mortality and re-revision following single-stage and two-stage revision surgery for the management of infected primary knee arthroplasty in England and Wales. Bone Joint Res. 2022;11:690–9.
6. Jackson WO, Schmalzried TP. Limited role of direct exchange arthroplasty in the treatment of infected total hip replacements. Clin Orthop Relat Res. 2000;381:101–5.
7. Zahar A, Kendoff DO, Klatte TO, Gehrke TA. Can good infection control be obtained in one-stage exchange of the infected TKA to a rotating hinge design? 10-year results. Clin Orthop Relat Res. 2016;474:81–7.
8. Aalirezaie A, Bauer TW, Fayaz H, et al. Hip and knee section, diagnosis, reimplantation: proceedings of international consensus on orthopedic infections. J Arthroplast. 2019;34:S369–79.
9. Gehrke T, Kendoff D. Peri-prosthetic hip infections: in favour of one-stage. Hip Int. 2012;22(Suppl 8):S40–5.
10. Segur JM, Vichez-Cavazos F, Martinez-Pastor JC, Macule F, Suso S, Acosta-Olivo C. Tibial tubercle osteotomy in septic revision total knee arthroplasty. Arch Orthop Trauma Surg. 2014;134:1311–5.
11. Fink B. Revision of late periprosthetic infections of total hip endoprostheses: pros and cons of different concepts. Int J Med Sci. 2009;6:287–95.
12. Göksan SB, Freeman MA. One-stage reimplantation for infected total knee arthroplasty. J Bone Joint Surg Br. 1992;74-B:78–82.
13. Tibrewal S, Malagelada F, Jeyasselan L, Posch F, Scott G. Single-stage revision for the infected total knee replacement: results from a single centre. Bone Joint J. 2014;96-B:759–64.
14. Hube R, Matziolis G, Kalteis T, Mayr HO. TKA revision of semiconstraint components using the 3-step technique. Oper Orthop Traumatol. 2011;23:61–9.
15. Fink B, Stefanou D. Three-step technique for implantation of rotating hinge knee prostheses: demonstration using the Enduro prosthesis. Oper Orthop Traumatol. 2020;32:329–39.
16. Hofmann AA, Goldberg TD, Tanner AM, Cook TM. Ten-year experience using an articulating antibiotic cement hip spacer for the treatment of chronically infected total hip. J Arthroplast. 2005;20:874–9.
17. Hoff SF, Fitzgerald RH, Kelly PJ. The depot administration of Penicillin G and gentamicin in acrylic bone cement. J Bone Joint Surg Am. 1981;63-A:789–804.
18. Cui Q, Mihalko WM, Shields JS, Ries M, Saleh HJ. Antibiotic-impregnated cement spacers for the treatment of infection associated with total hip or knee arthroplasty. J Bone Joints Surg Am. 2007;89-A:871–82.
19. Simpson PMS, Dall GF, Breusch SJ, Heisel C. In vitro elution and mechanical properties of antibiotic-loaded SmartSet HV and Palocor R acrylic bone cements. Orthopade. 2005;34:1255–62.
20. Baleani M, Persson C, Zolezzi C, Andollina A, Borelli AM, Tigani D. Biological and biomechanical effects of vancomycin and meropenem in acrylic bone cement. J Arthroplast. 2008;23:1232–8.

21. Anagnostakos K, Kelm J, Regitz T, Schmitt E, Jung W. In vitro elution of antibiotic release from and bacteria growth inhibition by antibiotic-loaded acrylic bone cement spacers. J Biomed Mater Res. 2005;72-B:373–8.
22. Ensing GT, van Horn JR, van der Mei HC, Busscher HJ, Neut D. Copal bone cement is more effective in preventing biofilm formation than Palacos R-G. Clin Orthop Relat Res. 2008;466:1492–8.
23. Penner MJ, Masri BA, Duncan CP. Elution characteristics of vancomycin and tobramycin combined in acrylic bone-cement. J Arhtroplasty. 1996;11:939–44.
24. Gehke T, Zahar A, Kendoff D. One-stage exchange: it all began here. Bone Joint J. 2013;95-B:77–83.
25. Salvati EA, Chekofsky KM, Braus BD, Wilson PD Jr. Reimplantation in infection: a 12-year experience. Clin Orthop Relat Res. 1982;170:62–75.
26. Tornford WW, Thongphasuk J, Mankin HJ, Ferrero MJ. Frozen musculoskeletal allografts: a study of the clinical incidence and causes of infection associated with their use. J Bone Joint Surg. 1990;72-A:1137–43.
27. Winkler H, Kaudela K, Stoiber A, Menschik F. Bone grafts impregnated with antibiotics as a tool for treating infected implants in orthopedic surgery—one stage revision results. Cell Tissue Bank. 2006;7:319–23.
28. Engh GA, Parks NL. The management of bone defects in revision total knee arthroplasty. Instr Course Lect. 1997;46:227–36.
29. Mancuso F, Beltrame A, Colombo E, Miani E, Bassini F. Management of metaphyseal bone loss in revision knee arthroplasty. Acta Biomed. 2017;88:98–111.
30. Reichel H, Hube R, Birke A, Hein W. Bone defects in revision total knee arthroplasty: classification and management. Zentralbl Chir. 2002;127:880–5.
31. Khan Y, Arora S, Kashyap A, Patralekh MK, Maini L. Bone defect classification in revision total knee arthroplasty, their reliability and utility: a systematic review. Arch Orthop Trauma Surg. 2023;143:453–68.
32. Rodriguez-Merchan EC, Gomez-Cardero P, Encinas-Ullan CA. Management of bone loss in revision total knee arthroplasty: therapeutic options and results. EFORT Open Rev. 2021;6:1073–86.
33. Patel JV, Masonis JL, Guerin J, Borne RB, Rorabeck CH. The fate of augments to treat type-2 bone defects in revision knee arthroplasty. J Bone Joint Surg. 2004;86-Br:195–9.
34. Boureau F, Putman S, Arnould A, Dereudre G, Migaud H, Pasquir G. Tantalum cones and bone defects in revision total knee arthroplasty. Orthop Traumatol Surg Res. 2015;101:251–5.
35. Burastero G, Cavagnaro L, Chiarlone F, Alessio-Mazzola M, Carrega G, Felli L. The use of tantalum metaphyseal cones for the management of severe bone defects in septic knee revision. J Arthroplast. 2018;33:3739–45.
36. Klim SM, Amerstorfer F, Bernhardt GA, Sadoghi P, Gruber G, Radl R, Leithner A, Glehr M. Septic revision total knee arthroplasty: treatment of metaphyseal bone defects using metaphyseal sleeves. J Arthroplast. 2018;33:3734–8.
37. Calori GM, Mazza EL, Vaienti L, Mazzola S, Colombo A, Gala L, Colombo M. Reconstruction of patellar tendon following implantation of proximal tibia megaprosthesis for the treatment of post-traumatic septic bone defects. Injury. 2016;47(Suppl 6):S77–82.
38. Smith EL, Shah A, Son SJ, Niu R, Talmo CT, Abdeen A, The Boston Arthroplasty Collaborative Megaprosthesis Writing Committee, Ali M, Pinski J, Gordon M, Lozano-Calderon S, Bedair HS. Survivorship of megaprostheses in revision hip and knee arthroplasty for septic and aseptic indications: a retrospective, multicenter study with minimum 2-year follow-up. Arthroplast Today. 2020;6:475–9.
39. Berend KR, Lombardi AV Jr. Distal femoral replacement in nontumor cases with severe bone loss and instability. Clin Orthop Relat Res. 2009;467:485–92.
40. Daines BK, Dennis DA. Management of bone defects in revision total knee arthroplasty. Instr Course Lect. 2013;62:341–8.
41. Citak M, Levent A, Suero EM, Rademacher K, Busch SM, Gehrke T. A novel radiological classification system of the distal femur. Arch Orthop Trauma Surg. 2022;142(2):315–22.

42. Linke P, Wilhelm P, Levent A, Gehrke T, Salber J, Akkaya M, Suero EM, Citak M. Anatomical risk factors for aseptic loosening of full hinge knee prosthesis in primary and revision TKAs. Arch Orthop Trauma Surg. 2023;143:4299–307.
43. Levent A, Suero EM, Gehrke T, Citak M. Risk factors for aseptic loosening after total knee arthroplasty with a rotating-hinge implant: a case-control study. J Bone Joint Surg Am. 2021;103:517–23.
44. Ohlmeier M, Alrustom F, Citak M, Rolvien T, Gehrke T, Frings J. The clinical outcome of different total knee arthroplasty designs in one-stage revision for periprosthetic infection. J Arthroplast. 2022;37:359–66.
45. Levent A, Suero EM, Gehrke T, Bakhtiari IG, Citak M. Risk factors for aseptic loosening in complex revision total knee arthroplasty using rotating hinge implants. Int Orthop. 2021;45:125–32.
46. Scholz T, Akkaya M, Linke P, Busch SM, Gehrke T, Salber J, Citak M. The anatomical shape of the distal femur is an independent risk factor for aseptic loosening following one-stage septic knee revision using rotating hinge knee prosthesis. Arch Orthop Trauma Surg. 2023;143:481–8.
47. Buller TL, Eccles CJ, Deckard ER, Ziemba-Davis M, Meneghini RM. The fate and relevance of the patella in two-stage revision total knee arthroplasty for periprosthetic joint infection. J Arthroplast. 2022;37:2090–6.
48. Tigani D, Trentani P, Trentani F, Andreoli I, Sabbioni G, Del Piccolo N. Trabecular metal patella in total knee arthroplasty with patella bone deficiency. Knee. 2009;16:46–9.
49. Nelson CL, Lonner JH, Lahiji A, Kim J, Lotke PA. Use of a trabecular metal patella for marked patella bone loss during revision total knee arthroplasty. J Arthroplasty. 2003;18(7 Suppl 1):37–41.
50. Scuderi C. Ruptures of the quadriceps tendon—study of twenty tendon ruptures. Am J Surg. 1958;95:626–35.
51. Chekofsky KM, Spero CR, Scott WN. A method of repair of late quadriceps rupture. Clin Orthop Relat Res. 1980;147:190–1.
52. Ecker ML, Lotke PA, Glazer RM. Late reconstructions of the patellar tendon. J Bone Joint Surg Am. 1979;61-A:884–6.
53. Vivacqua T, Moraes R, Barretto J, Cavanelas N, Albuquerque R, Mozella A. Functional outcome of patients undergoing knee arthrodesis after infected total arthroplasty. Rev Bras Ortop. 2021;56:320–5.
54. Troulliez T, Faure PA, Martinot P, Migaud H, Senneville E, Pasquier G, Dartus J, Putman S. Above-the-knee amputation versus knee arthrodesis for revision of infected total knee arthroplasty: recurrent infection rates and functional outcomes of 43 patients at a mean follow-up of 6.7 years. Orthop Traumatol Surg Res. 2021;107:102914.
55. Suda AJ, Cieslik A, Grützner PA, Münzberg M, Heppert V. Flaps for closure of soft tissue defects in infected revision knee arthroplasty. Int Orthop. 2014;38:1387–92.
56. Osei DA, Rebehn KA, Boyer MI. Soft-tissue defects after total knee arthroplasty: management and reconstruction. J Am Acad Orthop Surg. 2016;24:769–79.

HIP; Surgical Technique: Bone Loss and Muscle Insufficiency

Akos Zahar, Nandor J. Nemes, and Christian Lausmann

Periprosthetic joint infection (PJI) is a very challenging complication of total hip arthroplasty (THA) [1]. Despite all efforts to prevent this complication, infections occur in about 0.5–1.9% of primary hip arthroplasty and in 4–8% after revisions [2, 3]. Although the definitive diagnosis of PJI remains the key for success, a designated concept of preoperative planning and treatment is essential [1, 4, 5]. Treatment options include irrigation and debridement [6] with retention of implants for acute infections, or exchange arthroplasty for deep, late infections [7–11]. Where all reconstructive options fail, consideration is given to salvage operations, including a Girdlestone-like resection arthroplasty or disarticulation [7, 12]. Currently, "two-stage exchange" arthroplasty is the preferred method of treating chronic PJI of THA [13, 14], whereas a few specialized centers advocate protocol-based "one-stage exchange" arthroplasty with comparable outcomes [15–18].

The therapeutic goal in one-stage exchange arthroplasty is control of the infection combined with maintenance of joint function with a single surgery [16]. This technique is a viable option and should be used depending on the status of the patient [19], the surgeon's expertise, and the hospital set-up. The main objective is to reduce the bioburden by performing extensive and radical soft tissue debridement and removal of the biofilm-covered prosthesis.

On reviewing the current available literature and guidelines for the treatment of PJI [20], there is no clear evidence that two-stage exchange arthroplasty has a higher success rate than the one-stage approach [9]. Although the two-stage technique is described in many articles as the gold standard for management of chronic PJI [21],

A. Zahar (✉) · N. J. Nemes
St. George University Teaching Hospital, Szekesfehervar, Hungary
e-mail: azahar@mail.fmkorhaz.hu

C. Lausmann
Department of Orthopedic Surgery, Helios Endo-Klinik Hamburg, Hamburg, Germany

© The Author(s), under exclusive license to Springer Nature Switzerland AG 2024
M. Citak et al. (eds.), *One-Stage Septic Revision Arthroplasty*,
https://doi.org/10.1007/978-3-031-59160-0_6

there are several unknowns regarding this procedure; most importantly, optimal timing of the re-implantation [22].

The one-stage exchange offers some advantages, including the need for only one surgical procedure, reduced time on antibiotics, reduced hospital stay, and reduced overall costs [11]. Based on current evidence, the reported outcome of this procedure is comparable to two-stage exchange [18, 23–25], therefore one-stage exchange for PJI of THA is getting more popular worldwide. There is, however, a need for randomized prospective studies for direct comparison of the outcomes.

This article provides a detailed description of current practice regarding the management of PJI of the hip, including diagnostics, preoperative planning, surgical treatment algorithm, possible complications, and postoperative care.

One-Stage Exchange Arthroplasty

As described above, one-stage exchange arthroplasty carries many advantages compared with the two-stage exchange [16]. The former, though commonly performed in specialized centers in Europe, has also been gaining popularity in North America [26] and is a viable option for most patients with PJI [27]. At the Endo Klinik Hamburg, approximately 85% of patients with PJI are treated with one-stage exchange arthroplasty [5]. The main requirement for one-stage exchange arthroplasty is that the infecting organism and its sensitivity must be determined before surgery [28–30]. This allows for delivery of targeted local antibiotics, which are added to the cement [31, 32]. The indications and contraindications for one-stage septic exchange have been described in the chapter above.

Surgical Technique

The outcome of one-stage exchange arthroplasty is technique-dependent. This procedure largely depends on the efficiency by which debridement and bioburden reduction is performed. The technique of one-stage exchange arthroplasty is briefly outlined below.

Preoperative Planning

In every case, preoperative plain radiographs (anteroposterior and lateral views) are performed (Fig. 1a). In some difficult cases with massive bone loss, computed tomography (CT) imaging may be indicated. Preoperative templating using personal computer-based software (MediCAD, Hectec, Landshut, Germany) is done to reconstruct the proper leg-length, the lateral offset, and the center of rotation of the hip (see Fig. 1b). The proper implant sizes are templated and double-checked intraoperatively.

HIP; Surgical Technique: Bone Loss and Muscle Insufficiency

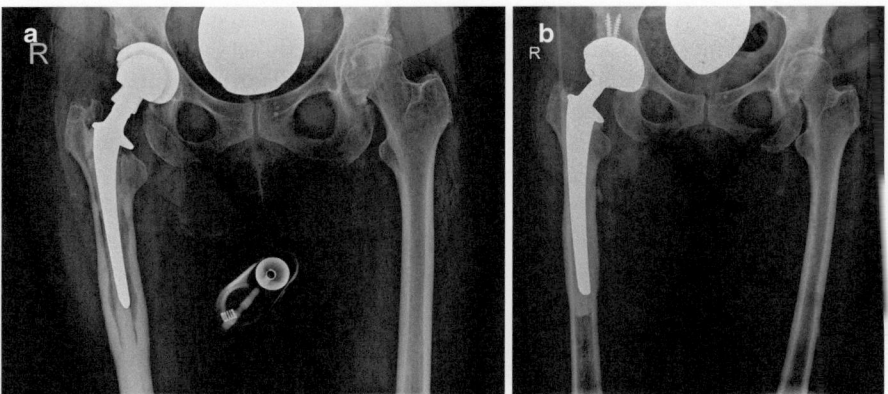

Fig. 1 (a) Preoperative ap radiograph of the pelvis with infected right total hip arthroplasty with cemented stem and cementless acetabular component. Extended head and taper section. Signs of osteolysis around the cup. Significant resorption of the cement around the stem with loosening. Femoral cortical thickening and medial cortical defect below the lesser trochanter. The contralateral side shows initial dysplastic hip arthritis. (b) Postoperative radiograph of the pelvis with hip arthroplasty on the right side. Acetabular reconstruction with Tantal revision shell fixed with two screws and cemented BiMobile Cup. Cemented stem fixation with slightly tubular palacos towards parossal soft tissue medially femoral via pre-existing small cortical defect

Preparation and Patient Positioning

Patients are placed in the lateral decubitus position with a well-fixed pelvis and with a special cushion between the legs providing a stable positioning with the affected leg freely moving in all planes. The skin is prepped 4 times with an alcoholic (propanol) solution (Cutasept G, Bode Chemie, Hamburg, Germany) with a minimum acting time of 2 min. Once the skin has dried, standard hip draping is performed with single-use materials. The length of incision and possible extension of the surgical approach should be considered so there is enough space for extensive surgical preparation.

Surgical Approach

The authors recommend a posterolateral approach to the infected hip, with old scars and draining sinuses integrated into the approach, if possible. Detachment of the maximus sling (attachment of the gluteus maximus muscle) allows for better access to the posterior aspect of the joint; moreover, the risk of sciatic nerve injury and periprosthetic femoral fracture (due to reduced rotational forces) is also reduced. With extra-articular preparation, the joint capsule is opened as late as possible to avoid contamination of the soft tissues. All capsule, synovia, and infective tissue are excised.

The advantage of the posterior approach is wide and unlimited access to all parts of the acetabulum and to the whole femur. Both endomedullary and periosteal preparation are easily performed. The approach can be extended to either direction; access to the distal part of the femur can be achieved by preparation along the intermuscular septum. Neurolysis of the sciatic nerve can be performed, if necessary. Positioning of both the acetabular and femoral components is reported to be safer and more reliable when using the posterolateral approach. The disadvantage of the approach is a reportedly higher risk of dislocation, although that can be avoided by proper positioning of the implants.

Surgical Procedure

Step 1. Debridement and Explantation

Debridement begins by excising the previous scar. The sinus, if present, should be integrated into the skin incision and radically excised down to the joint capsule [33]. All nonbleeding tissues and related bone need to be radically excised, and multiple tissue samples (4–6 for microbiology and 2 for pathohistology) are sent for further investigation [34, 35].

Special instruments are used for the removal of long and cemented stems, such as curved chisels, long forceps, curetting instruments, long drills, high-speed burrs, and cement taps (Fig. 2). Solid femoral implants may require a longitudinal osteotomy or, rarely, an extended trochanteric osteotomy. All implants, foreign material, cement, and restrictors need to be removed (Figs. 3 and 4). Generally, the debridement of bone and surrounding soft tissues must be as radical as possible and must include all areas of nonviable bone. Occasionally, resection of the greater trochanter or the proximal part of the femur is unavoidable, which necessitates the use of tumor-type, fully cemented, modular, long-stemmed revision implants and, sometimes, a higher level of constraint, such as a constrained liner or a dual mobility cup [11].

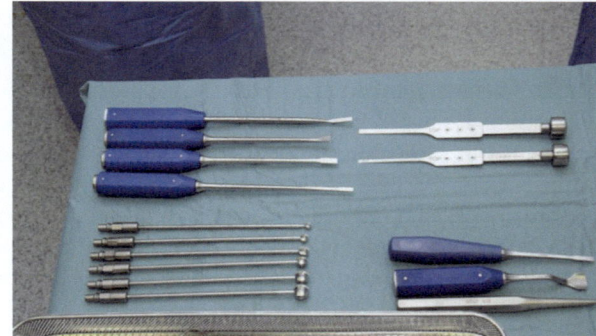

Fig. 2 Set of special chisels are needed to mobilize the solid implant in order to avoid femoral osteotomy. High-speed burrs facilitate the bone debridement and later the interdigitation of the new cement achieving good fixation for the new cemented implant

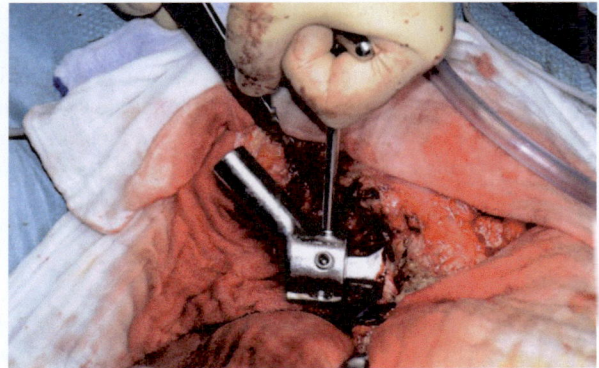

Fig. 3 A special explantation device is attached by drill holes (extra hard drill bit) and small screws to the metal taper of the solid implant, which is then removed by gliding mallet taps

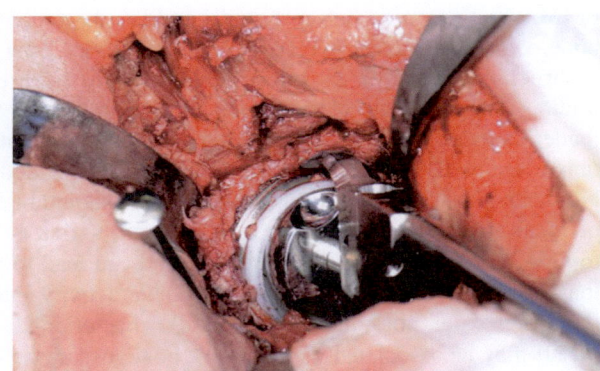

Fig. 4 Explantation instruments with sharp blades are used to cut out and mobilize the well-fixed uncemented acetabular component

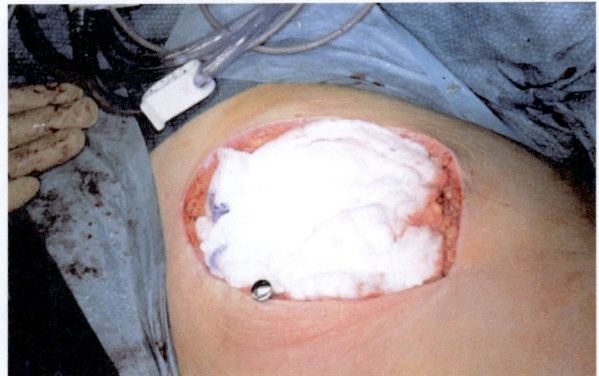

Fig. 5 The wound is packed with antiseptic-soaked towels and swabs for 10–15 min to achieve a high concentration of the antiseptic solution. Meanwhile a new draping is performed and a new set of instruments is used

Step 2. Irrigation with Local Antiseptics

The authors recommend the general use of pulsatile lavage throughout the procedure. After complete implant removal and debridement, the intramedullary canals are packed with polymeric biguanide hydrochloride (polyhexanide)-soaked swabs (Fig. 5). After the completion of resection, if the surgical site is considered clean, during the acting time (10–15 min) of the local antiseptic solution, a new surgical set-up is performed. This consists of rescrubbing by the surgeons, re-draping the surgical field, changing the suction tip and the light handles, and bringing new instruments for re-implantation. A complete new prepping of the patient is not possible because of the open wound. Intravenous antibiotics are given at this time according to the recommendation of the infectious disease specialist [31].

Step 3. Re-Implantation

Re-implantation may be performed with antibiotic-loaded cement which is prepared according to a strict protocol. This may contain water-soluble, heat-resistant antibiotics in crystalline form. The powder should be mixed with the powder of the PMMA bone cement before liquid is added. In general, manufactured antibiotic bone cements are used, such as Copal G + C or Copal G + V (Heraeus Medical, Wehrheim, Germany). However, according to the preoperative microbiological findings, an admixture of antibiotics may be indicated. When using the antibiotic-loaded cement for definitive fixation of a new implant during re-implantation, a maximum of 10% by weight antibiotic should be added to the cement to retain its biomechanical properties [36]. However, care should be taken with the total amount of local antibiotics used to prevent systemic toxicity. Although rarely described, topical antibiotics may be nephrotoxic and can lead to renal failure. It is essential that the antibiotic added to the cement (a) has activity against the infecting organism (b) is in powder, not liquid form, and (c) is bactericidal.

PJI may be associated with massive bone loss of the acetabular or femoral bone stock. In single-stage revision, bone stock must be restored at the time of the operation for the implant to properly engage in the bone. The authors prefer not to use allograft bone, although there have been favorable outcomes with the use of antibiotic-impregnated allografts [24, 37]. Acetabular defects can be restored with porous metal shells or augments, where the liner can be inserted with antibiotic-loaded bone cement, benefiting from the release of local antibiotics. Smaller defects may be filled with antibiotic-loaded polymethyl-methacrylate (PMMA) bone cement (Copal, Heraeus Medical, Hanau, Germany) [38]. On the femoral side, monoblock cemented stems are widely used (SPII Lubinus, Waldemar Link, Hamburg, Germany), while modular cemented (MP or Mega C modular systems, Waldemar Link, Hamburg, Germany) or uncemented revision stems are used in massive defects. Uncemeneted implants may be coated with an antimicrobial agent.

Septic revision may result in soft tissue destruction around the hip and gluteal insufficiency. In the posterior approach, repairing the capsule and external rotators (piriformis tendon) with non-absorbable sutures is a valuable option, although not always possible. With the trial heads on, one should perform the dislocation tests (combined flexion-adduction-internal rotation), the equator (or conplanar) test, and check for telescoping of the components to choose the appropriate head size ("the greater the better") and length. In case of instability, a retainment ring may be used. In addition, most implant companies now offer lipped (or anteverted) poly-liner options. The center of rotation should be determined during preoperative planning and restored during surgery to recreate the biomechanical environment of the hip. After implantation of THA in early postoperative period, abduction cushions may be used to prevent the patient from adducting the operated leg. In case of revisions with loss of the greater trochanter or insufficient gluteus medius, or after resection of the proximal femur, a dual mobility cup or a constrained cup should be considered. The dual mobility cup consists of a metal shell that encloses a movable polyethylene liner. The femoral head (diameter 22 or 28 mm) is encased by the hemispheric liner so that it also allows rotation of the femoral head within the polyethylene sphere. The polyethylene casing can articulate partly against the metal casing and partly against the femoral head fixed on the stem. The concept differentiates from the constrained liner used for uncemented cups, in which the insert is rigidly fixed in the metal shell. From a biomechanical perspective, a dual mobility system should have advantages compared to a constrained liner because extreme movements are not translated to shear force at the cup–bone interface. Moreover, proper offset selection is important to avoid impingement of the proximal femur or the femoral implant on the pelvis, which would make both systems unsafe.

Complications and Management

The persistence or recurrence of infection remains the most relevant complication following surgical intervention for PJI of the hip (Table 1). Failure rates with two-stage exchange range from 9% to 20% with non-resistant bacteria. Recently published data regarding one-stage septic exchange of the knee show comparable results for the one-stage exchange arthroplasty at short and midterm follow-up [18, 25, 39–45].

Table 1 Complications and actions following surgical intervention

Complication	Severity	Action
Wound healing problem	Mild	Early revision
Dislocation	Mild	Closed reduction
Repeated dislocation	Moderate	Open reduction, revision of components
Persistent infection	Severe	Early revision, exchange of modular components, debridement, reloading with local antibiotics
Failed single-stage exchange	Severe	Two-stage exchange with antibiotic spacer

Postoperative Care

Postoperative Antibiotics

In the one-stage approach, postoperative systemic antibiotic administration is usually continued for 10–14 days [31] through a central venous line. PJI with *Streptococci* may require a prolonged course of antibiotic therapy. After 2 weeks, IV administration may be switched to oral therapy depending on the resistance profile of the infecting organism [46]. The antibiotic therapy is determined by the infectious disease specialist, who is a member of the multidisciplinary team (MDT) involved in the whole diagnostic and therapy protocol of PJIs.

Physiotherapy

A major advantage of the one-stage technique is that patients can be ambulated early and allowed to start functional exercises. Due to the variety of soft tissue and bone damage and the extent of infection most cases require an individualized physiotherapy regime. Postoperative rehabilitation in these patients aims to reduce associated muscular movement restrictions, stiffness, or fibrosis of the affected hip joint. The authors generally recommend early mobilization within the first postoperative days using walking aids such as crutches. In most cases, full-weight bearing may be introduced immediately, whereas sometimes a more gradual approach is required over the first 2 weeks postoperatively based on intraoperative findings and substance defects.

Outcomes

The two-stage revision of PJI is considered to be the gold standard by most of the orthopedic surgeons [47], with a reported failure rate in terms of reinfection between 9% and 20%. By contrast, in our specialized hospital for bone and joint surgery, the authors have established and followed the one-stage approach described in this article for almost 40 years [5, 15]. There are good infection control rates for one-stage septic exchange of infected TKA and success is seen in about 90% of all our total joint arthroplasty patients at 10-year follow-up [39]. The results of one-stage septic exchange of THA are given in Table 2.

Far more studies have been published on the two-stage approach, and only a few studies have evaluated the one-stage exchange and its techniques in THA. However, these results show comparable success rates of 80–90%. Variations may result from different bacteria and follow-up times. As recent reports have shown, the overall results of two-stage revisions might have even higher complication and lower success rates than reported previously, especially with multiresistant organisms such as methicillin-resistant *Staphylococcus aureus* (MRSA) [48, 49].

Table 2 Summary of publications containing data about the infection control rate with one-stage septic exchange of total hip arthroplasty

Author	Year	Number of patients	Follow-up (years)	Infection control rate (%)
Wroblewski	1986	102	3.2	91
Loty et al.	1992	90	NA	91
Raut et al.	1995	183	7.8	84
Winkler et al.	2008	37	4.4	92
Klouche et al.	2012	38	2.0	100
Hansen et al.	2013	27	4.2	70
Choi et al.	2013	17	5.2	82
Zeller et al.	2014	157	5.0	95

In conclusion, while the two-stage exchange arthroplasty remains the gold standard for treating periprosthetic joint infections, the one-stage approach offers several advantages over two stage-exchange and shows promising results. With ongoing advancements and accumulating evidence, one-stage exchange may emerge as a viable alternative for selected patients, reducing the burden on patients and healthcare resources.

References

1. Fink B, Makowiak C, Fuerst M, Berger I, Schafer P, Frommelt L. The value of synovial biopsy, joint aspiration and C-reactive protein in the diagnosis of late peri-prosthetic infection of total knee replacements. J Bone Joint Surg Br. 2008;90:874–8.
2. Bozic KJ, Ries MD. The impact of infection after total hip arthroplasty on hospital and surgeon resource utilization. J Bone Joint Surg Am. 2005;87:1746–51.
3. Kurtz SM, Lau E, Schmier J, Ong KL, Zhao K, Parvizi J. Infection burden for hip and knee arthroplasty in the United States. J Arthroplast. 2008;23:984–91.
4. De Man FH, Sendi P, Zimmerli W, Maurer TB, Ochsner PE, Ilchmann T. Infectiological, functional, and radiographic outcome after revision for prosthetic hip infection according to a strict algorithm. Acta Orthop. 2011;82:27–34.
5. Gehrke T, Zahar A, Kendoff D. One-stage exchange: it all began here. Bone Joint J. 2013;95-B(11 Suppl A):77–83.
6. Romano CL, Manzi G, Logoluso N, Romano D. Value of debridement and irrigation for the treatment of periprosthetic infections. A systematic review. Hip Int. 2012;22(Suppl 8):S19–24.
7. Cierny G III, DiPasquale D. Periprosthetic total joint infections: staging, treatment, and outcomes. Clin Orthop Relat Res. 2002;403:23–8.
8. Hsieh PH, Shih CH, Chang YH, et al. Two-stage revision hip arthroplasty for infection: comparison between the interim use of antibiotic-loaded cement beads and a spacer prosthesis. J Bone Joint Surg Am. 2004;86-A:1989–97.
9. ICG. International Consensus Group on periprosthetic infection. Consensus statements. Philadelphia: Thomas Jefferson University; 2013.
10. Parvizi J, Adeli B, Zmistowski B, et al. Management of periprosthetic joint infection: the current knowledge: AAOS exhibit selection. J Bone Joint Surg Am. 2012;94:e104.
11. Zahar A, Webb J, Gehrke T, Kendoff D. One-stage exchange for prosthetic joint infection of the hip. Hip Int. 2015;25:301–7.

12. Haddad FS, Masri BA, Garbuz DS, Duncan CP. The treatment of the infected hip replacement. The complex case. Clin Orthop Relat Res. 1999;369:144–56.
13. Cooper HJ, Della Valle CJ. The two-stage standard in revision total hip replacement. Bone Joint J. 2013;95-B(11 Suppl A):84–7.
14. Engesaeter LB, Dale H, Schrama JC, et al. Surgical procedures in the treatment of 784 infected THAs reported to the Norwegian Arthroplasty Register. Acta Orthop. 2011;82:530–7.
15. Buchholz HW, Elson RA, Engelbrecht E, et al. Management of deep infection of total hip replacement. J Bone Joint Surg Br. 1981;63-B:342–53.
16. Gehrke T, Kendoff D. Peri-prosthetic hip infections: in favour of one-stage. Hip Int. 2012;22(Suppl 8):S40–5.
17. Steinbrink K, Frommelt L. Treatment of periprosthetic infection of the hip using one-stage exchange surgery. Orthopade. 1995;24:335–43. [in German].
18. Zeller V, Lhotellier L, Marmor S, et al. One-stage exchange arthroplasty for chronic periprosthetic hip infection: results of a large prospective cohort study. J Bone Joint Surg Am. 2014;96:e1.
19. McPherson EJ, Woodson C, Holtom P, et al. Periprosthetic total hip infection: outcomes using a staging system. Clin Orthop Relat Res. 2002;403:8–15.
20. Parvizi J, Della Valle CJ. AAOS clinical practice guideline: diagnosis and treatment of periprosthetic joint infections of the hip and knee. J Am Acad Orthop Surg. 2010;18:771–2.
21. Romano CL, Romano D, Albisetti A, et al. Preformed antibiotic-loaded cement spacers for two-stage revision of infected total hip arthroplasty. Long-term results. Hip Int. 2012;22(Suppl 8):S46–53.
22. Berend KR, Lombardi AV Jr, Morris MJ, et al. Two-stage treatment of hip periprosthetic joint infection is associated with a high rate of infection control but high mortality. Clin Orthop Relat Res. 2013;471:510–8.
23. Loty B, Postel M, Evrard J, et al. One stage revision of infected total hip replacements with replacement of bone loss by allografts. Study of 90 cases of which 46 used bone allografts. Int Orthop. 1992;16:330–8. [in French].
24. Winkler H, Stoiber A, Kaudela K, et al. One stage uncemented revision of infected total hip replacement using cancellous allograft bone impregnated with antibiotics. J Bone Joint Surg Br. 2008;90:1580–4.
25. Wroblewski BM. One-stage revision of infected cemented total hip arthroplasty. Clin Orthop Relat Res. 1986;211:103–7.
26. Jiranek WA, Waligora AC, Hess SR, et al. Surgical treatment of prosthetic joint infections of the hip and knee: changing paradigms? J Arthroplast. 2015;30:912–8.
27. Lichstein P, Gehrke T, Lombardi A, et al. One-stage vs two-stage exchange. J Arthroplast. 2014;29(Suppl 2):108–11.
28. Ince A, Rupp J, Frommelt L, et al. Is "aseptic" loosening of the prosthetic cup after total hip replacement due to nonculturable bacterial pathogens in patients with low-grade infection? Clin Infect Dis. 2004;39:1599–603.
29. Parvizi J, Ghanem E, Menashe S, et al. Periprosthetic infection: what are the diagnostic challenges? J Bone Joint Surg Am. 2006;88(Suppl 4):138–47.
30. Schinsky MF, Della Valle CJ, Sporer SM, et al. Perioperative testing for joint infection in patients undergoing revision total hip arthroplasty. J Bone Joint Surg Am. 2008;90:1869–75.
31. Frommelt L. Principles of systemic antimicrobial therapy in foreign material associated infection in bone tissue, with special focus on periprosthetic infection. Injury. 2006;37(Suppl 2):S87–94.
32. Hanssen AD, Spangehl MJ. Practical applications of antibiotic-loaded bone cement for treatment of infected joint replacements. Clin Orthop Relat Res. 2004;427:79–85.
33. Raut VV, Siney PD, Wroblewski BM. One-stage revision of infected total hip replacements with discharging sinuses. J Bone Joint Surg Br. 1994;76:721–4.
34. Krenn V, Morawietz L, Perino G, et al. Revised histopathological consensus classification of joint implant related pathology. Pathol Res Pract. 2014;210:779–86.

35. Schafer P, Fink B, Sandow D, et al. Prolonged bacterial culture to identify late periprosthetic joint infection: a promising strategy. Clin Infect Dis. 2008;47:1403–9.
36. Fink B, Vogt S, Reinsch M, et al. Sufficient release of antibiotic by a spacer 6 weeks after implantation in two-stage revision of infected hip prostheses. Clin Orthop Relat Res. 2011;469:3141–7.
37. Winkler H, Kaudela K, Stoiber A, et al. Bone grafts impregnated with antibiotics as a tool for treating infected implants in orthopedic surgery - one stage revision results. Cell Tissue Bank. 2006;7:319–23.
38. Schildhauer TA, Robie B, Muhr G, et al. Bacterial adherence to tantalum versus commonly used orthopedic metallic implant materials. J Orthop Trauma. 2006;20:476–84.
39. Zahar A, Kendoff DO, Klatte TO, et al. Can good infection control be obtained in one-stage exchange of the infected TKA to a rotating hinge design? 10-year results. Clin Orthop Relat Res. 2016;474:81–7.
40. Callaghan JJ, Katz RP, Johnston RC. One-stage revision surgery of the infected hip. A minimum 10-year followup study. Clin Orthop Relat Res. 1999;369:139–43.
41. Choi HR, Kwon YM, Freiberg AA, et al. Comparison of one-stage revision with antibiotic cement versus two-stage revision results for infected total hip arthroplasty. J Arthroplast. 2013;28(Suppl 8):66–70.
42. George DA, Konan S, Haddad FS, et al. Single-stage hip and knee exchange for periprosthetic joint infection. J Arthroplast. 2015;30:2264–70.
43. Hansen E, Tetreault M, Zmistowski B, et al. Outcome of one-stage cementless exchange for acute postoperative periprosthetic hip infection. Clin Orthop Relat Res. 2013;471:3214–22.
44. Klouche S, Leonard P, Zeller V, et al. Infected total hip arthroplasty revision: one- or two-stage procedure? Orthop Traumatol Surg Res. 2012;98:144–50.
45. Raut VV, Siney PD, Wroblewski BM. One-stage revision of total hip arthroplasty for deep infection. Long-term follow up. Clin Orthop Relat Res. 1995;321:202–7.
46. Kilgus DJ, Howe DJ, Strang A. Results of periprosthetic hip and knee infections caused by resistant bacteria. Clin Orthop Relat Res. 2002;404:116–24.
47. Wongworawat MD. Clinical faceoff: one- versus two-stage exchange arthroplasty for prosthetic joint infections. Clin Orthop Relat Res. 2013;471:1750–3.
48. Mortazavi SM, O'Neil JT, Zmistowski B, et al. Repeat 2-stage exchange for infected total hip arthroplasty: a viable option? J Arthroplast. 2012;27:923–6.e1.
49. Mortazavi SM, Vegari D, Ho A, et al. Two stage exchange arthroplasty for infected total knee arthroplasty: predictors of failure. Clin Orthop Relat Res. 2011;469:3049–54.

Shoulder: Surgical Technique, Complications, and Results

Philip Linke and Jörg Neumann

Introduction

Periprosthetic infection (PPI) in total shoulder arthroplasty (TSA) differs significantly from knee and hip arthroplasty. Even if the number of implantations is significantly lower in absolute terms, it will increase significantly with an estimated 90,000 TSA implantations per year in Germany by 2040. Consecutively, the number of revision arthroplasty procedures will also increase by a factor of 2.5–8.4 [1].

Up to now, there is a prevalence of approximately 0.4–4% after primary TSA [2] and up to 15% after revision TSA [3] for periprosthetic infection.

In a systematic review and meta-analysis, Seok et al. [4] showed that risk factors for the development of periprosthetic infection include previous non-arthroplasty surgery and male gender (Table 1).

The periprosthetic infection and its surgical consequences result in an increased mortality of up to 2.2 fold in comparison to aseptic revision surgery, independent of the surgical strategy (one versus two stage) [5].

In our experience, the classic classification as in hip and knee arthroplasty between early and late infection as well as acute or chronic infection is particularly important for the therapy decision as to whether it is still possible to retain the implanted arthroplasty (early infection, acute infection) [6]. In the case of a chronic infection, it can be assumed that the bacterium has already formed a biofilm [7] and that it is therefore no longer possible to retain the implants in order to eradicate the infection [8].

P. Linke · J. Neumann (✉)
Department of Orthopedic Surgery, Helios Endo-Klinik Hamburg, Hamburg, Germany
e-mail: joerg.neumann@helios-gesundheit.de

Table 1 Illustration of risk factors for periprosthetic infection, adapted from Seok et al. [4]

Risk factors	Odds Ratio
Demographic	
Male (sex)	1.71
ASA ≥ 3	0.87
Perioperative factors	
Previous surgery (non Arthroplasty)	2.4
Trauma diagnosis	1.74
Revision arthroplasty	0.21
Comorbidities	
Diabetes mellitus	1.32
Liver disease	1.7
Rheumatoid arthritis	1.59
Alcohol overuse	2.47
Iron-deficiency anemia	2.73

The otherwise frequently used classification according to acute (<3 months), subacute 3–12 months or chronic (> 12 months) after index surgery does not seem adequate in our opinion, as the onset of symptoms is not taken into account [9].

Furthermore, there is a controversy regarding the surgical therapy for PJI in TSA between one-stage and two-stage septic exchange [10]. In the two-stage exchange, the endoprosthesis is first explanted, radical debridement is performed and then a spacer is implanted. In a second operation, the spacer is explanted, radical debridement is performed again and the new prosthesis is reimplanted. In the time between the operations (usually 6 weeks), the patient is given oral antibiotics. With the spacer, only limited mobility and low weight-bearing can be achieved. This is the advantage of a one-time procedure. Radical debridement, explantation, and reimplantation are carried out in only one operation. In this way, the patient is exposed to only one operation with the associated perioperative risk. Historically, Prof. Buchholz, the founder of the ENDO Klinik, initiated the one-stage septic change in 1970. For the success of the one-stage septic change, it is important to consider certain points and requirements. In the following chapter, we explain the preparation, execution, and outcome of the one-stage septic change.

Diagnosis

Beyond the appropriate therapy, the diagnosis of periprosthetic joint infections (PJI) is one of the greatest challenges in shoulder arthroplasty. This is mainly due to an increased number of low-grade infections, which are usually associated with mild clinical symptoms and complicate the diagnosis [11].

A consistent definition with associated diagnostic criteria for TSA infection does not exist in the literature [12]. The 2018 ICM criteria, which are most commonly used in hip and knee arthroplasty, were adapted for shoulder surgery by Garrigues et al. [13, 14] and are largely based on the same parameters as the 2018 ICM criteria for hip and knee surgery [15].

A definite periprosthetic joint infection is determined according to the following criteria:

- Existence of a sinus tract.
- Macroscopic intraarticular pus.
- Two positive microbiological cultures with phenotypically identical virulent organism.

If these criteria are not given, the minor criteria for defining shoulder PJI are used (Table 2). It is important to differentiate which parameters can be assessed preoperatively and which can only be taken intraoperatively.

Table 2 Minor Criteria of adapted ICM 2018 [13]

Minor criteria	Weight
Unexpected wound drainage	4
Single positive tissue culture with virulent Organism	3
Single positive tissue culture with low-virulence Organism	1
Second positive tissue culture (identical Low-virulence organism)	3
Humeral loosening	3
Positive frozen section (5 PMNs in ≥5 High-power fields)	3
Positive preoperative aspirate culture (low or high virulence)	3
Elevated synovial neutrophil percentage (>80%)[a]	2
Elevated synovial WBC count (>3000 cells/μL)[a]	2
Elevated ESR (>30 mm/h)[a]	2
Elevated CRP level (>10 mg/L)[a]	2
Elevated synovial α-defensin level	2
Cloudy fluid	2

PJI periprosthetic joint infection, *PMN* polymorphonuclear leukocyte, *WBC* white blood Cee, *ESR* erythrocyte sedimentation rate, *CRP* C-reactive protein
[a]Beyond 6 weeks from recent surgery

The minor criteria have different weights, which are cumulatively calculated individually for each case and result in a score. A cumulatively calculated score of 6 or higher with simultaneously detected organism is described as probable PJI. If no germ was detected and there are also 6 or more points, it is a possible PJI. If there are 6 or fewer points, the following rules apply [13]

- Single positive culture with virulent organism indicates possible PJI.
- Two positive cultures with low-virulence organism indicates possible PJI.
- Negative cultures or only single positive culture with low-virulence organism indicates PJI unlikely.

However, the adapted ICM criteria of 2018 should also be critically evaluated. The classification of pathogens as low and high virulent is not clearly described. According to Unter Ecker [16] as well as Busch et al [17], a classification is described, the validity of which has not yet been investigated. In our opinion, a correct consideration of the frequently detected low virulent germs in infection TSA is not given here. Therefore, the virulence of the germ is not crucial in our clinical setting. Similarly, other parameters such as humeral loosening are so far without clinical evidence [14].

In order to determine the adapted ICM criteria 2018, besides radiological diagnostics (loosening signs) preoperative laboratory tests for infection parameters in serum (CRP, ESR) and in joint aspiration (white blood cell count (WBC), PMN %, α defensin) should be performed. For this purpose, it is absolutely necessary to perform a joint aspiration, which we strictly recommend, even if some of the literature does not attribute greater importance to this diagnostic method [18]. In accordance with the ENDO standard, a joint aspiration is performed in our hospital every time there is a suspicion of PJI and before every endoprosthetic revision surgery. Furthermore, all other joint replacements are aspirated if PJI is present, as a synchronous PJI can exist with a prevalence of 4% [19]. The joint aspiration should be cultured microbiologically for at least 14 days for possible bacterial detection [20]. In addition, no antibiotics should be given for an interval of at least 4 weeks prior to joint aspiration.

However, if preoperative diagnosis is unclear and PJI is still suspected, especially when no germ could be detected in the joint aspiration, we recommend a second joint aspiration. If the situation remains unclear, an open biopsy is indicated in our algorithm. Normally, a PJI can be identified in this way before a septic change procedure.

Concerning the germ spectrum, low virulent pathogens are more common in TSA with periprosthetic infection [11, 17], as already mentioned. Cutibacterium (formerly Propionibacterium) acnes is most frequently detected. Subsequently, coagulase-negative Staphylococci, Staph aures, and Streptococci are identified in

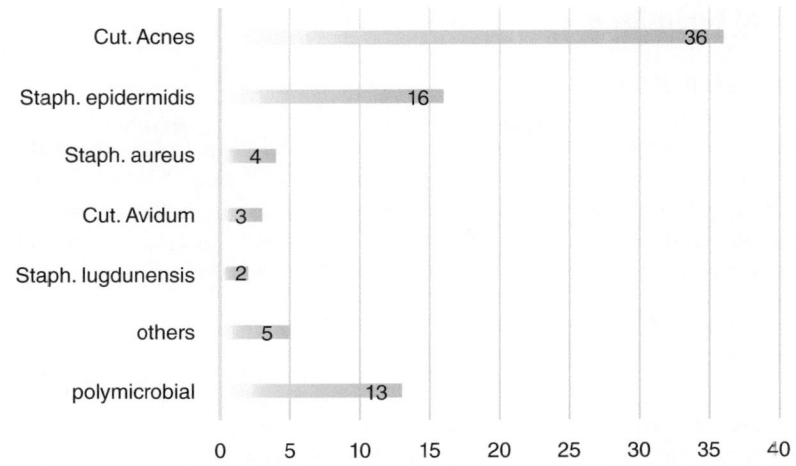

Fig. 1 Distribution of intraoperatively detected pathogens in our own collective (unpublished data)

microbiological diagnostics [10]. We also observed this distribution in our collective (Fig. 1).

However, not least because of the many different and inhomogeneous definitions of PJI in TSA, there is a high need for controlled studies on this topic.

Indications

As in knee and hip arthroplasty, the determining factor for success is the correct indication for a one-stage septic change. Furthermore, the identification of the germ is crucial for one-stage septic exchange and has the highest priority. The key to success in the diagnostic and surgery is also an interdisciplinary cooperation with infectious disease specialists and microbiologists, together with an accurate indication for one-stage or two-stage exchange.

The indication for a one-stage septic exchange is when a PJI with detection of the pathogen has been given. If a culture-negative PJI persists, specific antibiotic therapy is not possible and therefore a one-stage septic exchange should not be performed in this case. Similarly, two or more failed one-stage septic exchanges or sepsis are contraindications for a one-stage septic exchange. If there is intraoperative a high rate of infiltration of nerve-vessel bundles or if primary wound closure is not possible, a conversion to a two-stage procedure is indicated [21].

Surgical Technique

Preoperative Preparation

In addition to radiological diagnostics (Fig. 2a–c) and virtual planning of the new endoprosthetic component by means of computer software (MediCAD, Hectec, Landshut, Germany), the preparation for the surgery also includes the preparing of the systemic and local antibiotic therapy, which resulted from the interdisciplinary conference based on the microbiological findings and resistograms.

Approach

The patient is positioned in the beach chair position. Regarding the surgical approach, we recommend the deltopectoral approach independent of the primary approach to achieve sufficient exposure intraoperatively. Furthermore, excision of the old scar and, if present, excision of the sinus tract is performed (Fig. 3a, b). During preparation, collection of multiple biopsies for microbiological and histological diagnosis should be performed. Then, the humeral and glenoid components should be exposed and visualized (Fig. 4a–c).

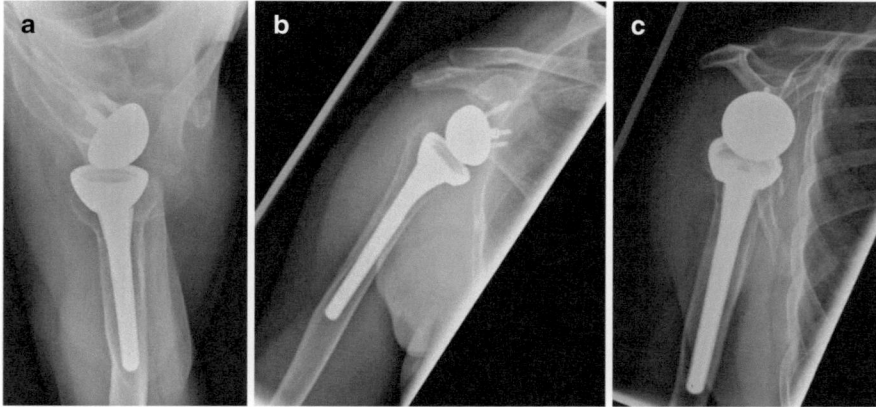

Fig. 2 (**a–c**) Preoperative radiological diagnostics with imaging of a reverse TSA with cementless fixation in case of proven periprosthetic infection in (**a**) axial, (**b**) true ap, and (**c**) y-view

Shoulder: Surgical Technique, Complications, and Results

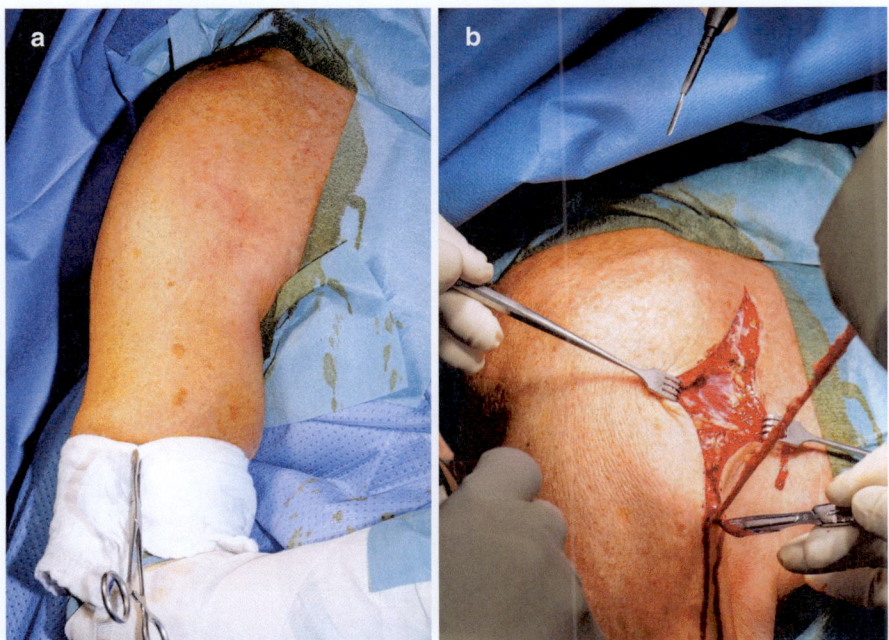

Fig. 3 (**a**, **b**): (**a**) Sterile draping, positioning in beach chair position; (**b**) Excision of the old scar of the deltopectoral approach

Explantation and Radical Debridement

Radical debridement with excision of the infected soft tissue should be carried out during the deep preparation. This also includes total synovectomy, especially of the dorsal part of the neo capsule (Fig. 5a–c). The explantation of the humeral and glenoid components is achieved with special instruments (Fig. 6a–c). It is crucial for the outcome that all foreign material is removed without exception and that the infected tissue is radically debrided. The cement remaining in the humeral canal after explantation should be removed with maximum caution to avoid iatrogenic perforation of the humeral shaft. When the debridement, which includes removal of infected soft tissue and bone (Fig. 7a–c), has been performed as radically as possible and the foreign material has been completely explanted, everything is extensively inflated with a pulsatile jet-lavage with biguanide-hydrochloride (polyhexanide) solution (Fig. 8a, b). Afterwards, we recommend changing the instruments to new or uncontaminated ones, as well as replacing the gloves, light handles, and the superficial drape.

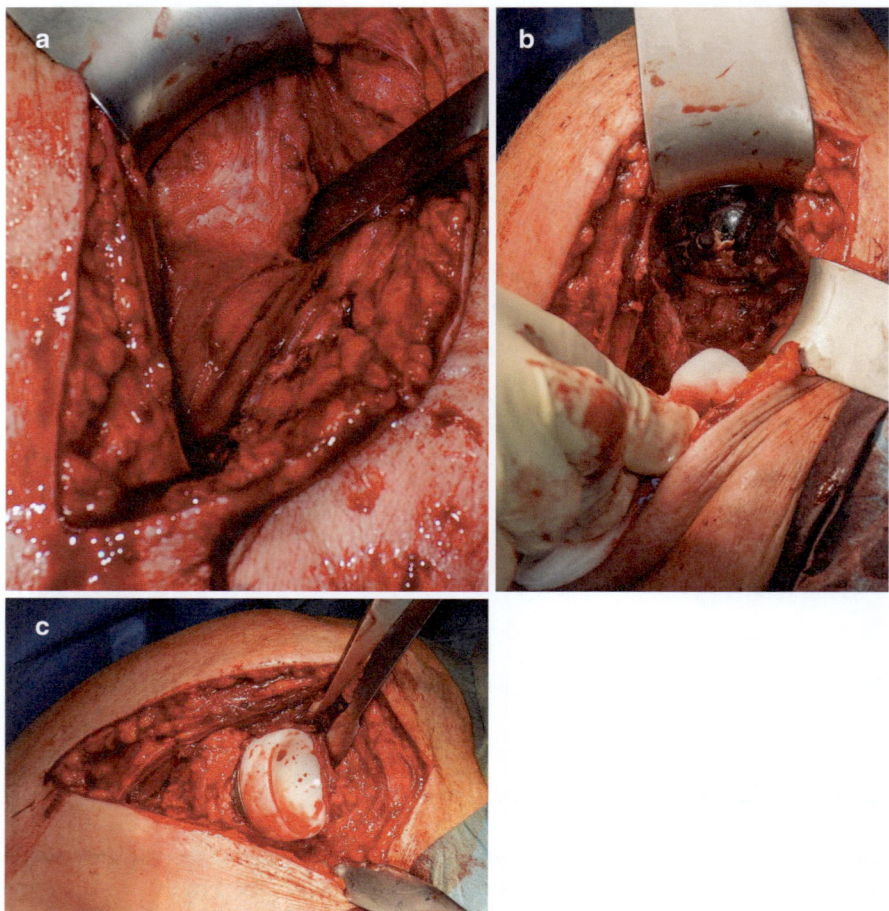

Fig. 4 (**a**–**c**) Visualisation of the situs with (**a**) infectious membrane over the glenosphere; (**b**) and after superficial debridement; (**c**) Visualization of the humeral tray after superficial debridement

Reimplantation

After radical debridement, intravenous antibiotics can be started. For the humeral component we strictly recommend choosing a cemented fixation in order to additionally provide a local antibiotic therapy. The use of bone allografts in the context of septic exchange should be avoided and existing defects should be reconstructed with antibiotic-loaded polymethyl methacrylate (PMMA) bone cement (Copal, Heraeus Medical, Hanau, Germany) as possible (Fig. 9). Nevertheless, it is necessary in some cases, especially for glenoid reconstruction. In the majority of cases, another antibiotic (often vancomycin) is added to this cement. It should be noted that the addition of an antibiotic to an existing PMMA bone cement combination causes a change in the polymerization behavior of the bone cement [22] (Fig. 10).

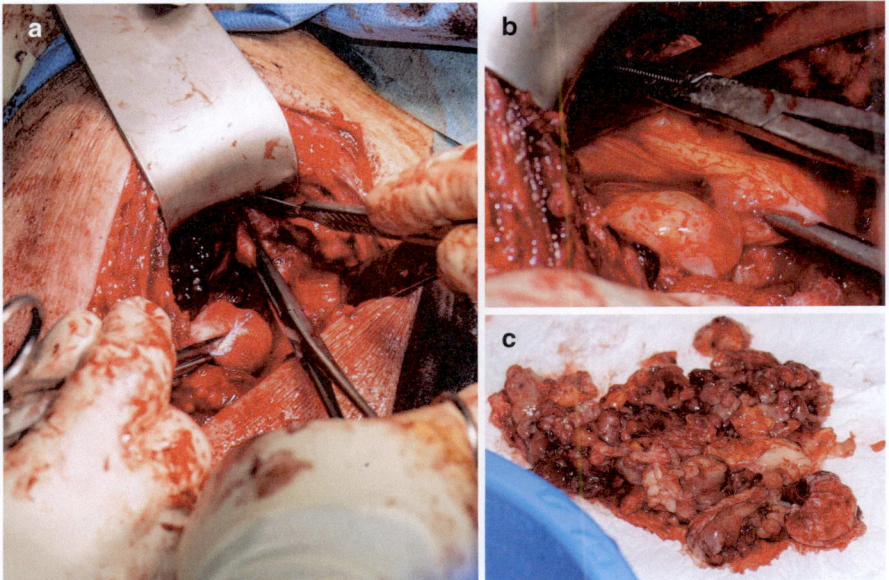

Fig. 5 (a–c) Radical debridement (a) of the labrum glenoidale with parts of the superoventral capsule; (b) of the dorsal capsule; (c) resected infected soft tissue

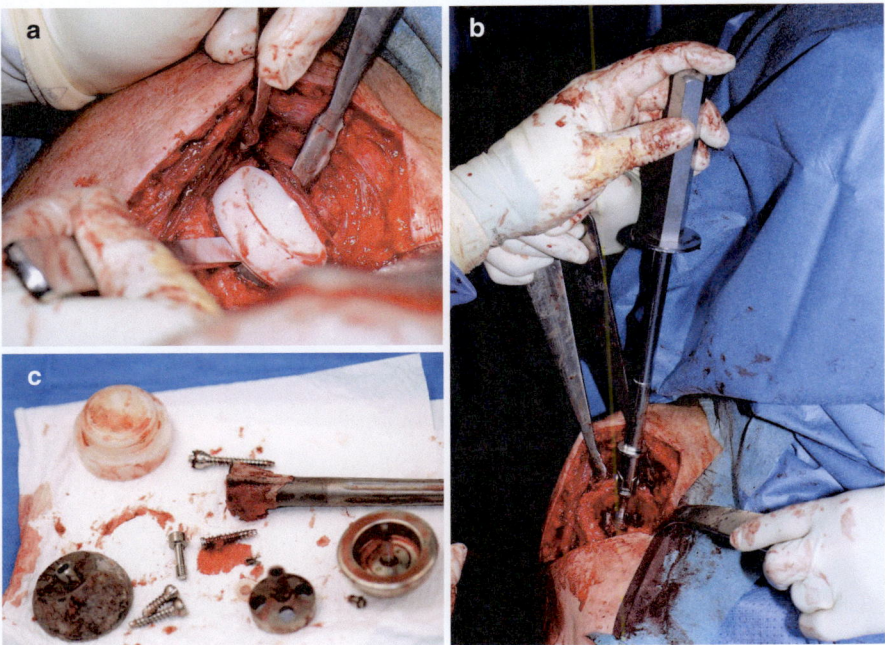

Fig. 6 (a–c): (a) Explantation of the humeral tray with a chisel; (b) Removal instrument for the humeral stem component; (c) Visualization of the completely removed prosthetic material

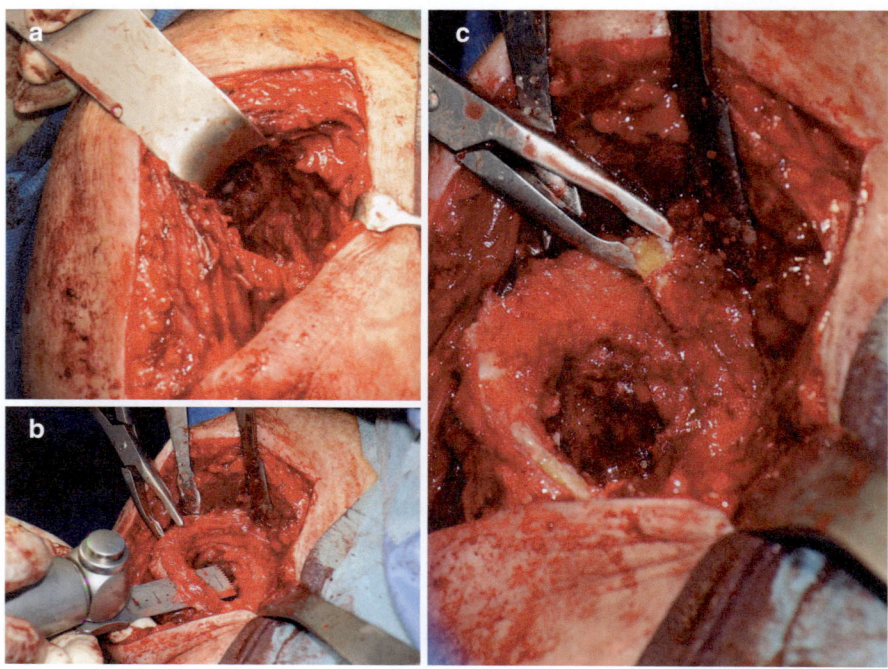

Fig. 7 (a–c): (a) Cavitas glenoidale after radical debridement; (b) Removal of osteomyelitic parts of the proximal humerus with the bone saw; (c) Radical bone debridement

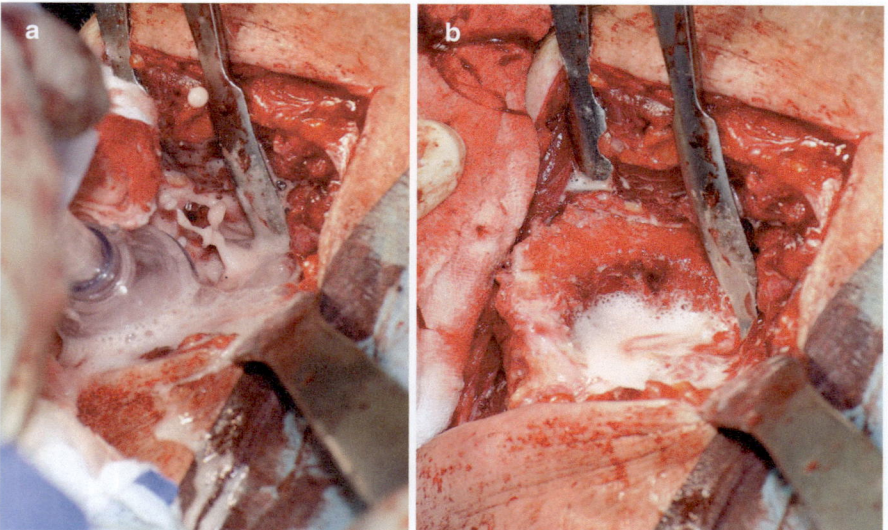

Fig. 8 (a, b): Jet-lavage with biguanide-hydrochloride (polyhexanide) solution

Shoulder: Surgical Technique, Complications, and Results

Fig. 9 Reimplantation of the humeral component with reconstruction after bone loss at the proximal humerus using PMMA bone cement

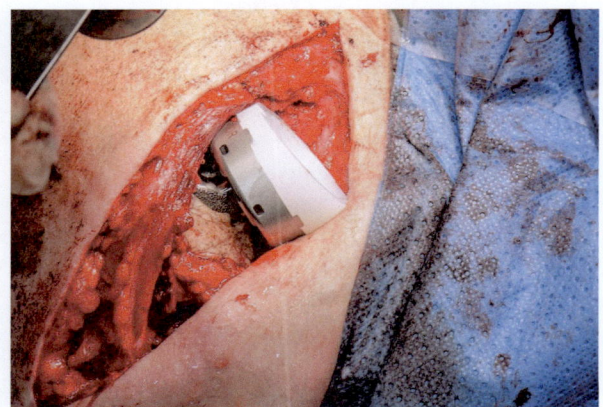

Fig. 10 Sterile manual addition of an antibiotic to an existing PMMA bone cement combination

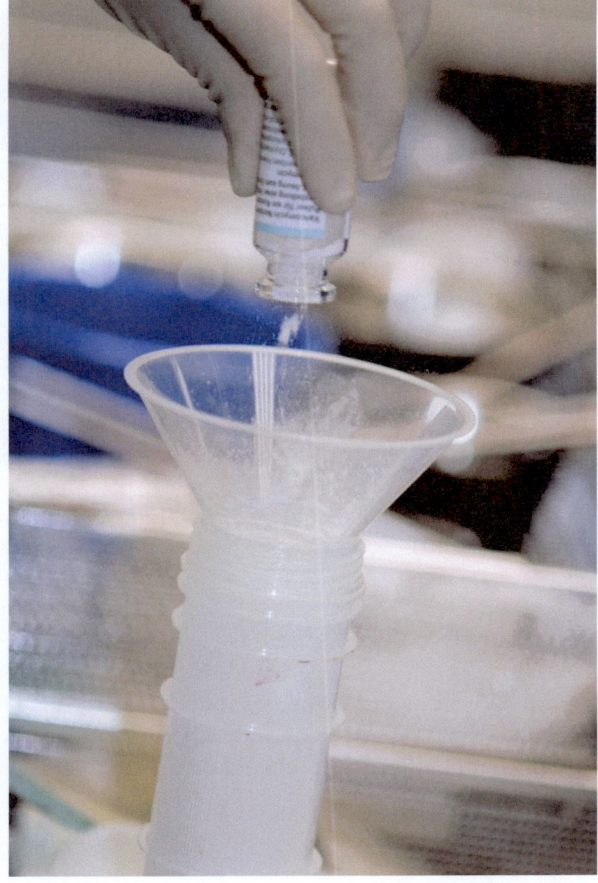

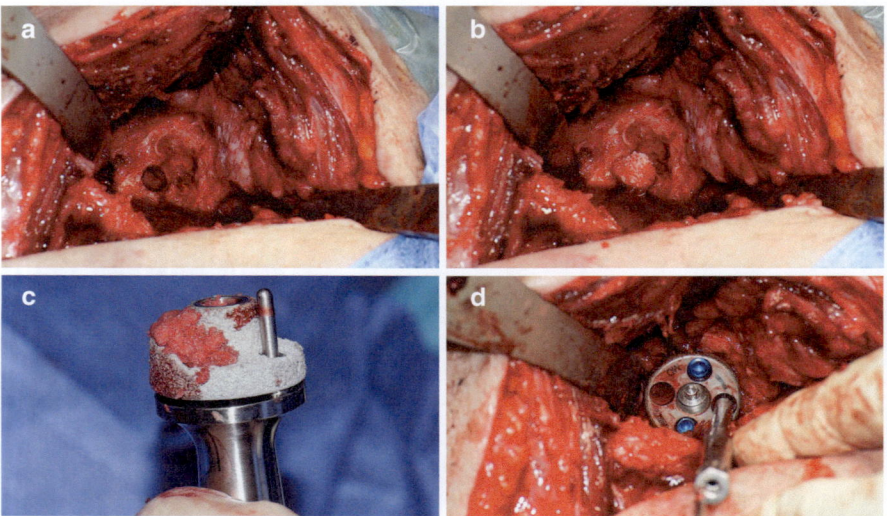

Fig. 11 (**a–d**): (**a**) Visualization of the glenoid after radical debridement with (**b**) addition of allogeneic spongiosa; (**c**) metal back augmented glenoid baseplate with additional allogeneic spongiosaplasty; (**d**) after implantation of augmented baseplate

In septic shoulder surgery, glenoid reconstruction is particularly challenging. Reimplantation with anatomical TSA is not recommended due to radical debridement with total synovectomy and severe loss of the rotator cuff. If the glenoid defect is mild, reconstruction with a normal or by severe defect with metal-augmented base plate is recommended. In addition, the glenoid and humeral eccentric options should be used to achieve sufficient lateralization and distalization (Fig. 11a–d). However, after debridement, the glenoid defect is often too large and so the bone defect is massive, a bipolar prosthesis must be implanted. In these cases, the glenoid can be reconstructed in a second procedure and the bipolar prosthesis can be converted to an inverse TSA.

Finally, the wound should be closed in layers and a suction drainage is recommended (Fig. 12).

Postoperative Care

Postoperative imaging should be routinely performed to verify the position of the implanted material and to exclude a periprosthetic fracture (Fig. 13). The limb is initially immobilized in a close-fitting orthosis. The inserted drain is removed

Fig. 12 Closed wound with indwelling suction drainage

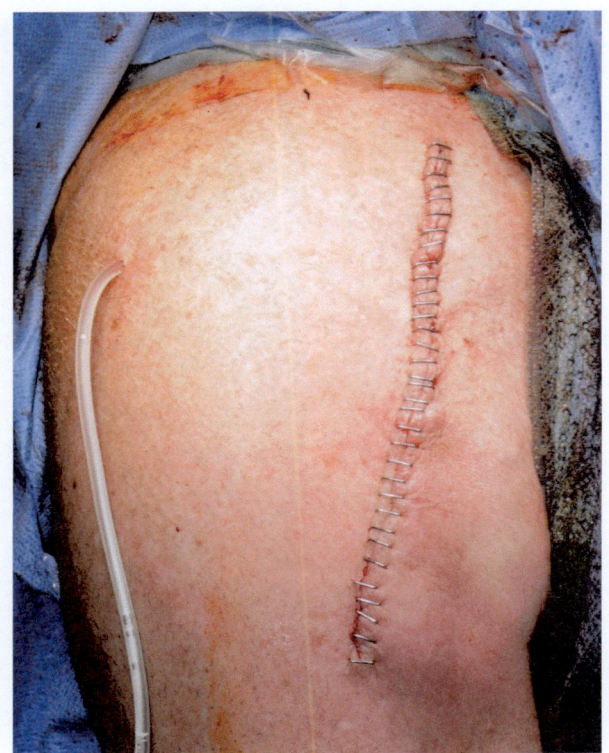

after 48 h and the tip of the drain is preserved under sterile conditions for microbiological diagnosis. The post-treatment regime starts with only passive mobilization for the first 2 weeks and begins with active-assistive movement from the third week postoperatively. Systemic antibiotic therapy should be individually adapted and in most cases administered intravenously for at least 14 days. For this purpose, a central venous catheter is inserted in every patient with a septic intervention at our hospital.

The patient is discharged from the inpatient setting after intravenous therapy. Subsequently, oral antibiotic sequential therapy should be continued for another 6 weeks. Here, the recommendation of the infectious disease specialists regarding the resistogram and the availability of the oral antibiotic should be considered.

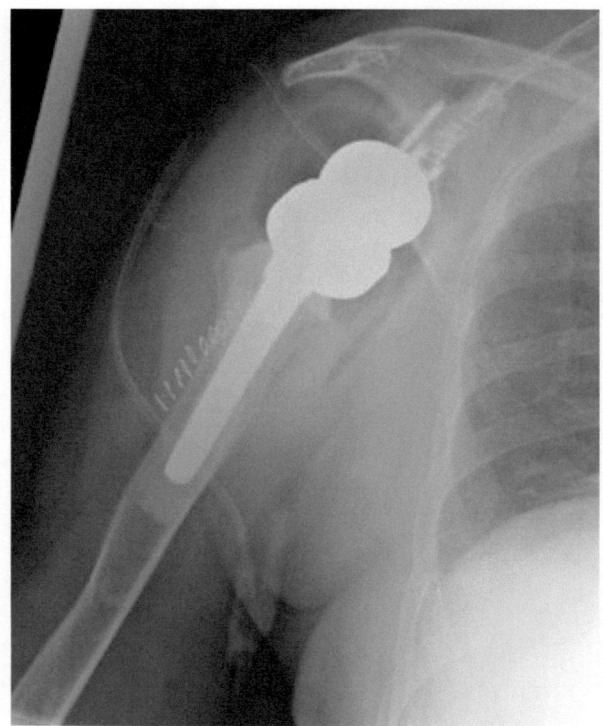

Fig. 13 Postoperative imaging after one-stage septic exchange with reimplantation of reverse TSA with an augmented baseplate

Complications

Reinfection is one of the most severe complications, as it is associated with treatment failure. The high eradication rates published in our institution [23, 24] have also been shown in other studies. For example, in a systematic review by Belay et al. [10], a reinfection rate of 6.3% after single-stage and 10.1% after two-stage septic exchange was described. Similarly, another review shows an overall infection clearance rate of 95.6% for one-stage and 85.2% for two-stage procedures [25].

Other complications include postoperative hematoma, perioperative fracture, instability, and nerve injury. The overall complication rate after one stage was lower (11.4%) than after two stages (22.5%) [10]. Compared to other surgical techniques such as DAIR and resection arthroplasty, the one-stage septic exchange also has a comparatively low complication rate of 11% [26].

Mercurio et al. [26] also described in their systemic review a low revision rate of 6% after one stage compared to two stage (15%).

Results

Although the eradication of infection is the primary outcome for surgeons in septic surgery, experience has shown that patients are more likely to want a high functional outcome. The data on clinical outcome scores are limited. Overall, the literature shows a good postoperative outcome after one stage with an expected Constant Score of 52.9 on average, which is similar to that after two-stage septic exchange (51.8) [10].

However, some studies describe a significant restriction of the range of motion (ROM) postoperatively [10]. This is probably due to the frequently implanted bipolar prostheses, especially after one-stage septic exchange. In our experience, patients manage well with a bipolar prosthesis related to daily activities and rarely need a conversion to reverse TSA.

In the systematic review by Mercurio et al. [26], besides the patient-reported outcome measurements (PROMs), there was no significant difference in ROM.

Overall, there is a comparable outcome after one-stage septic exchange with at least the same high eradication rate than two-stage exchange.

References

1. Klug A, Herrmann E, Fischer S, Hoffmann R, Gramlich Y. Projections of primary and revision shoulder arthroplasty until 2040: facing a massive rise in fracture-related procedures. J Clin Med. 2021;10(21):5123. https://doi.org/10.3390/jcm10215123.
2. Mook WR, Garrigues GE. Diagnosis and management of periprosthetic shoulder Infections. J Bone Joint Surg Am. 2014;96(11):956–65. https://doi.org/10.2106/JBJS.M.00402.
3. Grosso MJ, Frangiamore SJ, Yakubek G, Bauer TW, Iannotti JP, Ricchetti ET. Performance of implant sonication culture for the diagnosis of periprosthetic shoulder infection. J Shoulder Elb Surg. 2018;27(2):211–6. https://doi.org/10.1016/j.jse.2017.08.008.
4. Seok HG, Park JJ, Park SG. Risk factors for Periprosthetic joint infection after shoulder arthroplasty: systematic review and meta-analysis. J Clin Med. 2022;11(14):4245. https://doi.org/10.3390/jcm11144245.
5. Austin DC, Townsley SH, Rogers TH, Barlow JD, Morrey ME, Sperling JW, et al. Shoulder Periprosthetic joint infection and all-cause mortality: a worrisome association. JB JS Open Access. 2022;7(1):e21.00118. https://doi.org/10.2106/JBJS.OA.21.00118.
6. Tsukayama DT, Goldberg VM, Kyle R. Diagnosis and management of infection after total knee arthroplasty. J Bone Joint Surg Am. 2003;85-A(Suppl 1):S75–80. https://doi.org/10.2106/00004623-200300001-00014.
7. Hall-Stoodley L, Costerton JW, Stoodley P. Bacterial biofilms: from the natural environment to infectious diseases. Nat Rev Microbiol. 2004;2(2):95–108. https://doi.org/10.1038/nrmicro821.
8. Gehrke T, Alijanipour P, Parvizi J. The management of an infected total knee arthroplasty. Bone Joint J. 2015;97-B(10 Suppl A):20–9. https://doi.org/10.1302/0301-620X.97B10.36475.
9. Sperling JW, Kozak TK, Hanssen AD, Cofield RH. Infection after shoulder arthroplasty. Clin Orthop Relat Res. 2001;382:206–16. https://doi.org/10.1097/00003086-200101000-00028.

10. Belay ES, Danilkowicz R, Bullock G, Wall K, Garrigues GE. Single-stage versus two-stage revision for shoulder periprosthetic joint infection: a systematic review and meta-analysis. J Shoulder Elb Surg. 2020;29(12):2476–86. https://doi.org/10.1016/j.jse.2020.05.034.
11. Updegrove GF, Armstrong AD, Kim HM. Preoperative and intraoperative infection workup in apparently aseptic revision shoulder arthroplasty. J Shoulder Elb Surg. 2015;24(3):491–500. https://doi.org/10.1016/j.jse.2014.10.005.
12. Hsu JE, Somerson JS, Vo KV, Matsen FA 3rd. What is a "periprosthetic shoulder infection"? A systematic review of two decades of publications. Int Orthop. 2017;41(4):813–22. https://doi.org/10.1007/s00264-017-3421-6.
13. Garrigues GE, Zmistowski B, Cooper AM, Green A, Group ICMS. Proceedings from the 2018 international consensus meeting on orthopedic infections: the definition of periprosthetic shoulder infection. J Shoulder Elb Surg. 2019;28(6S):S8–S12. https://doi.org/10.1016/j.jse.2019.04.034.
14. Garrigues GE, Zmistowski B, Cooper AM, Green A, Group ICMS. Proceedings from the 2018 international consensus meeting on orthopedic infections: evaluation of periprosthetic shoulder infection. J Shoulder Elb Surg. 2019;28(6S):S32–66. https://doi.org/10.1016/j.jse.2019.04.016.
15. Shohat N, Bauer T, Buttaro M, Budhiparama N, Cashman J, Della Valle CJ, et al. Hip and knee section, what is the definition of a periprosthetic joint infection (PJI) of the knee and the hip? Can the same criteria be used for both joints?: proceedings of international consensus on orthopedic infections. J Arthroplast. 2019;34(2S):S325–S7. https://doi.org/10.1016/j.arth.2018.09.045.
16. Unter Ecker N, Suero EM, Gehrke T, Haasper C, Zahar A, Lausmann C, et al. Serum C-reactive protein relationship in high—versus low-virulence pathogens in the diagnosis of periprosthetic joint infection. J Med Microbiol. 2019;68(6):910–7. https://doi.org/10.1099/jmm.0.000958.
17. Busch SM, Citak M, Akkaya M, Prange F, Gehrke T, Linke P. Risk factors for mortality following one-stage septic hip arthroplasty—a case-control study. Int Orthop. 2021;46:507. https://doi.org/10.1007/s00264-021-05230-y.
18. Jauregui JJ, Tran A, Kaveeshwar S, Nadarajah V, Chaudhri MW, Henn RF 3rd, et al. Diagnosing a periprosthetic shoulder infection: a systematic review. J Orthop. 2021;26:58–66. https://doi.org/10.1016/j.jor.2021.07.012.
19. Thiesen DM, Mumin-Gunduz S, Gehrke T, Klaber I, Salber J, Suero E, et al. Synchronous Periprosthetic joint infections: the need for all artificial joints to be aspirated routinely. J Bone Joint Surg Am. 2020;102(4):283–91. https://doi.org/10.2106/JBJS.19.00835.
20. Schafer P, Fink B, Sandow D, Margull A, Berger I, Frommelt L. Prolonged bacterial culture to identify late periprosthetic joint infection: a promising strategy. Clin Infect Dis. 2008;47(11):1403–9. https://doi.org/10.1086/592973.
21. Zahar A, Gehrke TA. One-stage revision for infected Total hip arthroplasty. Orthop Clin North Am. 2016;47(1):11–8. https://doi.org/10.1016/j.ocl.2015.08.004.
22. Citak M, Luck S, Linke P, Gehrke T, Kuhn KD. Manual addition of antibiotics to industrial bone cement mixes : investigations of the dry mix in the cement cartridge during manual admixture to polymer-active substance mixtures. Orthopade. 2021;51:44. https://doi.org/10.1007/s00132-021-04115-7.
23. Ince A, Seemann K, Frommelt L, Katzer A, Loehr JF. One-stage exchange shoulder arthroplasty for peri-prosthetic infection. J Bone Joint Surg Br. 2005;87(6):814–8. https://doi.org/10.1302/0301-620X.87B6.15920.
24. Klatte TO, Junghans K, Al-Khateeb H, Rueger JM, Gehrke T, Kendoff D, et al. Single-stage revision for peri-prosthetic shoulder infection: outcomes and results. Bone Joint J. 2013;95-B(3):391–5. https://doi.org/10.1302/0301-620X.95B3.30134.
25. Ruditsky A, McBeth Z, Curry EJ, Cusano A, Galvin JW, Li X. One versus 2-stage revision for shoulder arthroplasty infections: a systematic review and analysis of treatment selection bias. JBJS Rev. 2021;9(9):1. https://doi.org/10.2106/JBJS.RVW.20.00219.
26. Mercurio M, Castioni D, Ianno B, Gasparini G, Galasso O. Outcomes of revision surgery after periprosthetic shoulder infection: a systematic review. J Shoulder Elb Surg. 2019;28(6):1193–203. https://doi.org/10.1016/j.jse.2019.02.014.

Fungal Periprosthetic Joint Infection

Mustafa Akkaya, Serhat Akcaalan, and Mustafa Citak

Introduction

Periprosthetic joint infection (PJI) is the most difficult complication after joint replacement. PJI is a complication that occurs in 0.7–2% of all arthroplasty cases, negatively affecting the quality of life, and sometimes even fatal [1]. The causative bacterial strains (50–60% Staf.aureus and Coagulase-negative staphylococci) were detected in 98% of PJI [2]. Although PJI cases caused by fungi are very rare with 1–2%, there are difficulties in treatment and management due to the lack of a consistent algorithm in the literature [2]. The increasing aging population and the increase in the immunosuppressed population have caused an increase in the incidence of periprosthetic fungal infections over time [3]. Fungal pathogens are mostly seen as causative microorganisms in immunosuppressive hosts, in patients who have received long-term antibiotic therapy, and in patients with a history of multiple surgeries [3]. However, diagnosis of fungal PJI is difficult because may be more difficult compared with bacterial pathogens because of diverse clinical presentations [4]. Surgical and medical management of fungal periprosthetic infections is more difficult than gram-positive or negative infections because these patients are mostly immunosuppressed, and the risk of persistent infection is higher. Although there is increasing interest in the diagnosis and management of bacterial PJI, there is not yet a standard guideline for fungal periprosthetic joint infections [4]. It takes a long time to isolate by traditional culture methods, and some of the culture-negative PJIs are thought to be due to fungi. Many centers often prefer two-stage revision surgery for fungal PJI treatment. However, some fungal strains are quite

M. Akkaya · S. Akcaalan · M. Citak (✉)
Department of Orthopedic Surgery, Helios Endo-Klinik Hamburg, Hamburg, Germany
e-mail: mustafa@drakkaya.com; mustafa.citak@helios-gesundheit.de

resistant to treatment and many patients are faced with treatment outcomes leading to arthrodesis, lifelong spacer retention, suppressive medical therapy, and even amputation [5, 6]. In this section, a detailed evaluation given with the current literature on fungal PJI.

Diagnosis in Fundal PJI

The diagnosis process of patients with fungal periprosthetic joint infection should begin with a detailed medical history and physical examination, as in all PJI patients. The surgeries that the patient has undergone, the complications that occur in the post-surgical period, the length of hospital stay and comorbid diseases should be questioned. If fungal PJI is suspected after this medical history; IV drug dependence, immunosuppression, long-term antibiotic use, systemic corticosteroid use, etc., which are predisposing factors for fungal PJI such cases should also be questioned in detail. Because these predisposing factors are encountered in at least 50% of the patients who develop fungal PJI. Some studies have shown that the incidence of predisposing factors in fungal PJI cases is much higher than 50% [7, 8].

Unlike bacterial infections, fungal PJI tends to present as chronic pain without erythema, swelling or effusion [7–9]. Fungal microorganisms are slow-growing pathogens that produce a biofilm that escapes the body's immune response. Fungi are very difficult to isolate in culture. Therefore, the diagnosis is delayed and they are diagnosed as chronic infection. Systemic symptoms such as fever and malaise are not very common in cases of fungal PJI [10].

The Musculoskeletal Infection Society and International Consensus Meeting recommended the diagnosis of PJI by considering clinical findings, serological and synovial biomarkers, and histological analysis [11]. Serum biomarkers are the first tests used when PJI is suspected.

According to the American Academy of Orthopedic Surgeons (AAOS) Clinical Practice Guidelines, the first laboratory tests in patients with a painful prosthesis and suspected PJI should start with erythrocyte sedimentation rate (ESR) and C-Reactive Protein (CRP). However, studies with these biomarkers are mostly based on the diagnosis of bacterial PJI. It is not known exactly whether the cut-off values determined in bacterial PJIs are valid in fungal PJIs. In the literature, it was determined that there were very different ESR and CRP values in the studies evaluated by patients with fungal PJI [8, 10, 12]. In meta-analyses evaluating fungal PJI cases, it was shown that only 50% of fungal PJI patients had elevated ESR and CRP [7, 9]. In patients with suspected PJI, aspiration may be required for synovial fluid analysis and culture. Since synovial markers provide a more specific evaluation, they are still frequently preferred in the diagnosis of PJI. Especially the WBC count and %PMN ratio in the synovial fluid are very valuable in diagnosing PJI. However, there is not much information about their validity and reliability in fungal PJI. Synovial leukocyte esterase, which is used in the diagnosis of bacterial PJI, cannot be used in fungal PJI. Because unlike bacteria, leukocyte esterase activity of fungal microorganisms cannot be measured [13].

Identification of the pathogen is very important for diagnosing fungal PJI and determining the treatment plan. However, in approximately 46% of fungal PJIs, the culture may be negative due to the difficulty of isolating the pathogenic organism [14]. Fungi have a slow growth pattern, therefore, fungal cultures should be incubated for at least 5–14 days, and in doubtful cases this incubation period should be extended to 4 weeks [8, 9]. Synovial fluid cultures can be used in blood culture bottles to increase the possibility of fungal isolation [15].

The most frequently isolated pathogen in fungal PJI cases is Candida species. C. Albicans was isolated in 47% of the cases, followed by C. parapsilosis and C. glabrata. More rarely isolated Candida species include C. pelliculosa and guilliermondii. Of the fungal pathogens isolated in fungal PJI cases, only 12% are non-Candida species. The most common non-Candida species are Aspergillus spp., Pichia anomala, and Coccidioides immitis. Apart from these pathogens, fungal PJI cases in various mycoses may rarely be causative pathogens [16].

Treatment

There is no consensus on the surgical treatment of fungal PJI. In the case of fungal PJI, retention of the prosthesis is nearly difficult, and a two-stage exchange is recommended [8, 17–19]. Studies in the literature show the success rate of two-state septic exchanges from fungal PJI treatment between 47% and 100% [8, 20]. The mean time between the two stages in fungal PJI was found to be 5.8 months [16]. In the first stage of two-stage septic exchange, prosthesis removal and spacer application are performed. Spacer applications in bacterial PJIs typically use a combination of vancomycin and gentamicin, or an antipseudomonal agent such as piperacillin or amikacin. However, antifungal agents such as amphotericin B and voriconazole are used in spacer applications in fungal PJIs [16]. However, there is no clear consensus on the dosages of these anti-fungals. The success rates of patients treated using antifungal spacers differ in the literature. In the literature, cure races were reported as 57% and 63% in two different studies [5, 21]. However, there are studies in the literature reporting a higher success rate than these studies using antifungal spacers [22, 23].

One-stage septic exchange has gained popularity in Europe and is being implemented in more and more centers. One state septic exchange enables PJI treatment with less morbidity, mortality, and cost. However, in order to apply one state septic exchange, patients must comply with some selective criteria. These are the identification of the causative microorganism in the pre-operative process, the absence of soft tissue loss, the patient's non-immunosuppressive and susceptibility to bactericidal treatment [24]. For these reasons, it was thought that the role of one state septic exchange applications in fungal PJI may be limited. Because the majority of fungal PJI patients have problems with the immune system. However, there are surgeons in the literature who have achieved a successful success rate as a result of one state septic exchange applied in cases of fungal PJI. Darouiche and Cardinal performed one state septic exchange in hip fungal PJI and stated that re-infection did not occur [7]. Azzam et al. applied joint debridement as a treatment instead of septic exchange; however, they encountered up to 75% re-infection [8]. Herndon et al., which has the largest cohort of fungal PJI in the literature, shared the treatment results in fungal PJI cases in their study; they stated that treatment failure rates are high in fungal PJI and that much more studies are needed to develop these treatment modalities [25].

Although combined antifungal therapy is strongly recommended in addition to surgical treatment, there is no clear consensus in the literature about the agent to be used. In patients infected with candida species, Pappas et al. recommend the use of fluconazole and echinocandins [26], and Parvizi et al. recommend the use of fluconazole or any amphotericin B [27]. When examined in other studies in the literature, the widespread use of both azoles and amphotericin B has been reported [28–31]. However, while Amphotericin B was used as the first choice antifungal in the 1980s–1990s, the use of azoles has become more widespread since the 2000s. There is no consensus in the literature regarding the duration of antifungal treatment in fungal PJIs. Parvizi et al. recommended 6 weeks of treatment [27], other studies in the literature argue that long-term treatment should be continued [17, 32, 33]. In addition, 6–12 months of use in chronic cases has been positively associated with treatment success [17]. It is stated in the literature that patients need a minimum follow-up period of 1 year for the success of fungal PJI treatment [34].

References

1. Beam E, Osmon D. Prosthetic joint infection update. Infect Dis Clin N Am. 2018;32:843–59. https://doi.org/10.1016/J.IDC.2018.06.005.
2. Tande AJ, Patel R. Prosthetic joint infection. Clin Microbiol Rev. 2014;27:302–45. https://doi.org/10.1128/CMR.00111-13.
3. Koutserimpas C, Chamakioti I, Zervakis S, Raptis K, Alpantaki K, Kofteridis DP, et al. Non-Candida fungal prosthetic joint infections. Diagnostics (Basel). 2021;11:11. https://doi.org/10.3390/DIAGNOSTICS11081410.
4. Nace J, Siddiqi A, Talmo CT, Chen AF. Diagnosis and management of fungal periprosthetic joint infections. J Am Acad Orthop Surg. 2019;27:e804–18. https://doi.org/10.5435/JAAOS-D-18-00331.
5. Brown TS, Petis SM, Osmon DR, Mabry TM, Berry DJ, Hanssen AD, et al. Periprosthetic joint infection with fungal pathogens. J Arthroplast. 2018;33:2605–12. https://doi.org/10.1016/J.ARTH.2018.03.003.
6. Hwang BH, Yoon JY, Nam CH, Jung KA, Lee SC, Han CD, et al. Fungal peri-prosthetic joint infection after primary total knee replacement. J Bone Joint Surg Br. 2012;94:656–9. https://doi.org/10.1302/0301-620X.94B5.28125.
7. Schoof B, Jakobs O, Schmidl S, Klatte TO, Frommelt L, Gehrke T, et al. Fungal periprosthetic joint infection of the hip: a systematic review. Orthop Rev (Pavia). 2015;7:18–22. https://doi.org/10.4081/OR.2015.5748.
8. Azzam K, Parvizi J, Jungkind D, Hanssen A, Fehring T, Springer B, et al. Microbiological, clinical, and surgical features of fungal prosthetic joint infections: a multi-institutional experience. J Bone Joint Surg Am. 2009;91(Suppl 6):142–9. https://doi.org/10.2106/JBJS.I.00574.
9. Jakobs O, Schoof B, Klatte TO, Schmidl S, Fensky F, Guenther D, et al. Fungal periprosthetic joint infection in total knee arthroplasty: a systematic review. Orthop Rev (Pavia). 2015;7:7. https://doi.org/10.4081/OR.2015.5623.

10. Geng L, Xu M, Yu L, Li J, Zhou Y, Wang Y, et al. Risk factors and the clinical and surgical features of fungal prosthetic joint infections: a retrospective analysis of eight cases. Exp Ther Med. 2016;12:991–9. https://doi.org/10.3892/ETM.2016.3353.
11. Parvizi J, Gehrke T. Definition of periprosthetic joint infection. J Arthroplast. 2014.29:1331. https://doi.org/10.1016/J.ARTH.2014.03.009.
12. Klatte TO, Junghans K, Al-Khateeb H, Rueger JM, Gehrke T, Kendoff D, et al. Single-stage revision for peri-prosthetic shoulder infection: outcomes and results. Bone Joint J. 2013;95-B:391–5. https://doi.org/10.1302/0301-620X.95B3.30134.
13. Kauffman CA, Fisher JF, Sobel JD, Newman CA. Candida urinary tract infections—diagnosis. Clin Infect Dis. 2011;52(Suppl):6. https://doi.org/10.1093/CID/CIR111.
14. Yoon HK, Cho SH, Lee DY, Kang BH, Lee SH, Moon DG, et al. A review of the literature on culture-negative periprosthetic joint infection: epidemiology, diagnosis and treatment. Knee Surg Relat Res. 2017;29:155–64. https://doi.org/10.5792/KSRR.16.034.
15. Geller JA, MacCallum KP, Murtaugh TS, Patrick DA, Liabaud B, Jonna VK. Prospective comparison of blood culture bottles and conventional swabs for microbial identification of suspected periprosthetic joint infection. J Arthroplast. 2016;31:1779–83. https://doi.org/10.1016/J.ARTH.2016.02.014.
16. Gross CE, Della Valle CJ, Rex JC, Traven SA, Durante EC. Fungal Periprosthetic joint infection: a review of demographics and management. J Arthroplasty. 2021;36:1758–64. https://doi.org/10.1016/J.ARTH.2020.11.005.
17. Ueng SWN, Lee CY, Hu CC, Hsieh PH, Chang Y. What is the success of treatment of hip and knee candidal periprosthetic joint infection? Clin Orthop Relat Res. 2013;471:3002–9. https://doi.org/10.1007/S11999-013-3007-6.
18. Wang QJ, Shen H, Zhang XL, Jiang Y, Wang Q, Chen YS, et al. Staged reimplantation for the treatment of fungal peri-prosthetic joint infection following primary total knee arthroplasty. Orthop Traumatol Surg Res. 2015;101:151–6. https://doi.org/10.1016/J.OTSR.2014.11.014.
19. Kuiper JWP, Van Den Bekerom MPJ, Van Der Stappen J, Nolte PA, Colen S. 2-stage revision recommended for treatment of fungal hip and knee prosthetic joint infections. Acta Orthop. 2013;84:517–23. https://doi.org/10.3109/17453674.2013.859422.
20. Anagnostakos K, Kelm J, Schmitt E, Jung J. Fungal periprosthetic hip and knee joint infections clinical experience with a 2-stage treatment protocol. J Arthroplast. 2012;27:293–8. https://doi.org/10.1016/J.ARTH.2011.04.044.
21. Gao Z, Li X, Du Y, Peng Y, Wu W, Zhou Y. Success rate of fungal Peri-prosthetic joint infection treated by 2-stage revision and potential risk factors of treatment failure: a retrospective study. Med Sci Monit. 2018;24:5549–57. https://doi.org/10.12659/MSM.909168.
22. Skedros JG, Keenan KE, Updike WS, Oliver MR. Failed reverse Total shoulder arthroplasty caused by recurrent Candida glabrata infection with prior Serratia marcescens coinfection. Case Rep Infect Dis. 2014;2014:1–9. https://doi.org/10.1155/2014/142428.
23. Escolà-Vergé L, Rodríguez-Pardo D, Lora-Tamayo J, Morata L, Murillo O, Vilchez H, et al. Candida periprosthetic joint infection: a rare and difficult-to-treat infection. J Infect. 2018;77:151–7. https://doi.org/10.1016/J.JINF.2018.03.012.
24. Gehrke T, Zahar A, Kendoff D. One-stage exchange: it all began here. Bone Joint J. 2013;95-B:77–83. https://doi.org/10.1302/0301-620X.95B11.32646.
25. Herndon CL, Rowe TM, Metcalf RW, Odum SM, Fehring TK, Springer BD, et al. Treatment outcomes of fungal Periprosthetic joint infection. J Arthroplast. 2023;38:2436. https://doi.org/10.1016/J.ARTH.2023.05.009.
26. Pappas PG, Kauffman CA, Andes DR, Clancy CJ, Marr KA, Ostrosky-Zeichner L, et al. Clinical practice guideline for the management of candidiasis: 2016 update by the Infectious Diseases Society of America. Clin Infect Dis. 2016;62:e1–50. https://doi.org/10.1093/CID/CIV933.
27. Parvizi J, Gehrke T, Chen AF. Proceedings of the international consensus on periprosthetic joint infection. Bone Joint J. 2013;95-B:1450–2. https://doi.org/10.1302/0301-620X.95B11.33135.
28. Younkin S, Evarts CM, Steigbigel RT. Candida parapsilosis infection of a total hip-joint replacement: successful reimplantation after treatment with amphotericin B and 5-fluorocytosine. A case report. J Bone Joint Surg Am. 1984;66:142–3.

29. Dumaine V, Eyrolle L, Baixench MT, Paugam A, Larousserie F, Padoin C, et al. Successful treatment of prosthetic knee Candida glabrata infection with caspofungin combined with flucytosine. Int J Antimicrob Agents. 2008;31:398–9. https://doi.org/10.1016/J.IJANTIMICAG.2007.12.001.
30. Ramamohan N, Zeineh N, Grigoris P, Butcher I. Candida glabrata infection after total hip arthroplasty. J Infect. 2001;42:74–6. https://doi.org/10.1053/JINF.2000.0763.
31. Hennessy MJ. Infection of a total knee arthroplasty by Candida parapsilosis. A case report of successful treatment by joint reimplantation with a literature review. Am J Knee Surg. 1996;9:133–6.
32. Phelan DM, Osmon DR, Keating MR, Hanssen AD. Delayed reimplantation arthroplasty for candidal prosthetic joint infection: a report of 4 cases and review of the literature. Clin Infect Dis. 2002;34:930–8. https://doi.org/10.1086/339212.
33. Saconi ES, De Carvalho VC, De Oliveira PRD, Lima ALLM. Prosthetic joint infection due to Candida species: case series and review of literature. Medicine. 2020;99:E19735. https://doi.org/10.1097/MD.0000000000019735.
34. Belden K, Cao L, Chen J, Deng T, Fu J, Guan H, et al. Hip and knee section, fungal periprosthetic joint infection, diagnosis and treatment: proceedings of international consensus on orthopedic infections. J Arthroplast. 2019;34:S387–91. https://doi.org/10.1016/J.ARTH.2018.09.023.

Management of Reinfection After One-Stage Exchange Arthroplasty

Gerard A. Sheridan, Michael E. Neufeld, Andrea Volpin, and Bassam A. Masri

Introduction

Reinfection after one-stage exchange arthroplasty for PJI is a failure to achieve the goal of treatment and represents a challenging clinical problem for both clinicians and patients alike. With the increasing popularity of one-stage exchange for PJI, reinfection in this patient population is a problem surgeons will be faced with more in the future. Although studies in the last few years have been published reporting on this patient population, the literature remains quite limited.

The risks of one-stage exchange failure in the hip have been investigated and reported by Abdelaziz et al. [1]. In their cohort of 121 patients, all patients underwent an initial single-stage exchange hip arthroplasty procedure for PJI, which was then followed by subsequent revision. The commonest causes of revision were instability (44%) followed by reinfection (33%) and aseptic loosening (13%). In that cohort, the factors associated with reinfection after initial single-stage exchange (including both new and persistent infections) were prolonged wound drainage (OR, 6.9; 95% CI, 2.2–21.5; $p = 0.001$) and prior surgery due to infection (OR, 4.3; 95% CI, 1.9–9.5; $p < 0.001$). These findings emphasize the need for meticulous wound closure when performing a single-stage exchange and an awareness of the risk posed by the patient having had prior procedures to manage infection.

The risks of one-stage exchange failure in the knee have also been reported by Citak et al. [2]. Ninety-one TKA patients were reported as undergoing revision following a single-stage exchange for PJI management in the knee. Eleven

G. A. Sheridan · M. E. Neufeld · B. A. Masri (✉)
Department of Orthopaedics, University of British Columbia, Vancouver, BC, Canada
e-mail: sheridga@tcd.ie; michael.neufeld@vch.ca; Bas.masri@vch.ca

A. Volpin
NHS Grampian, Aberdeen, UK

© The Author(s), under exclusive license to Springer Nature Switzerland AG 2024
M. Citak et al. (eds.), *One-Stage Septic Revision Arthroplasty*,
https://doi.org/10.1007/978-3-031-59160-0_9

variables were associated with reinfection after single-stage exchange as follows: weight > 100 kg, DVT, > 4 procedures, polymicrobial infection, preceding one-stage exchange due to PJI, preceding two-stage exchange due to PJI, surgery time > 4 h, persistent wound drainage, wound revision due to healing disorders, isolation of Streptococcus species and isolation of Enterococcus species. When using binary logistic regression analysis, there were four factors associated with reinfection: history of one-stage exchange, history of two-stage exchange, Enterococci species isolation, and Streptococci species isolation ($p = 0.013$).

On occasion, the principles of single-stage exchange demand complete eradication of infection with extensive debridement of infected bone stock. For the control of infection in the hip, a proximal femoral replacement may need to be performed. Abdelaziz reported on 57 patients undergoing proximal femoral replacement (PFR) for infection control as part of a single-stage revision procedure for PJI [3]. Although PFR may be required to remove all infected bones, when compared to controls, PFR increases both the all-cause rate of revision (29.8% vs. 10.%, $p = 0.018$) and especially the risk of revision due to reinfection (15.8% vs. 0%, $p = 0.003$).

Having considered the factors that increase the risk of reinfection in patients after single-stage exchange for PJI, we will now review the surgical treatment options for patients who have failed single-stage exchange due to reinfection.

Debridement, Antibiotics, Implant Retention (DAIR)

There is utility in debridement, antibiotics, and implant retention (DAIR) in the context of revision arthroplasty for recurrent prosthetic joint infection (PJI) [4, 5]. Performing a DAIR procedure allows the surgeon to retain hardware, and therefore reduce operative time, minimize bone loss, and lessen the surgical morbidity that the patient endures. A recent study by Veerman et al. analyzed the results of a DAIR procedure for infection within 90 days of revision total hip arthroplasty (rTHA) or revision total knee arthroplasty (rTKA) in 88 patients [6]. Overall, DAIR eradicated infection and resulted in retained hardware in 68% of the cohort at 2 years. Predictors of poor outcomes included an interval of greater than 30 days between rTHA/rTKA and DAIR, a repeat DAIR within 90 days and the use of immunosuppressant agents.

DAIR procedures are particularly useful in the setting of extensive hardware where complete removal of all well-fixed implants would lead to massive bone loss, thereby significantly limiting patient function and complicating any further surgery that the patient may undergo. A recent study by Barry et al. examined the results of 87 patients with PJI and extensive instrumentation [4]. Fifty-six patients were managed with DAIR and suppression whereas 31 patients were managed with 2-stage exchange. Re-operation for infection was 37.5% in the DAIR group and 32.3% in the 2-sage exchange group ($p = 0.62$). Only 41.9% of the 2-stage group underwent reimplantation and did not require further surgery compared to 62.5% in the DAIR group that did not require further surgery. Although this study did not compare 2-stage exchange to DAIR after a 1-stage exchange arthroplasty, the principle still applies supporting DAIR as a good option for infection control, particularly in the context of extensive hardware, which would be present in many patients who have undergone a single-stage exchange arthroplasty.

Although there are no specific studies analyzing the effectiveness of DAIR after a 1-stage exchange arthroplasty, there is good evidence supporting the use of DAIR after revision THA and TKA, especially in the context of extensive hardware, as it reduces infection recurrence and increases the likelihood of implant retention. Figures 1 and 2 demonstrate a case of DAIR procedures after a failed single-stage exchange due to PJI recurrence.

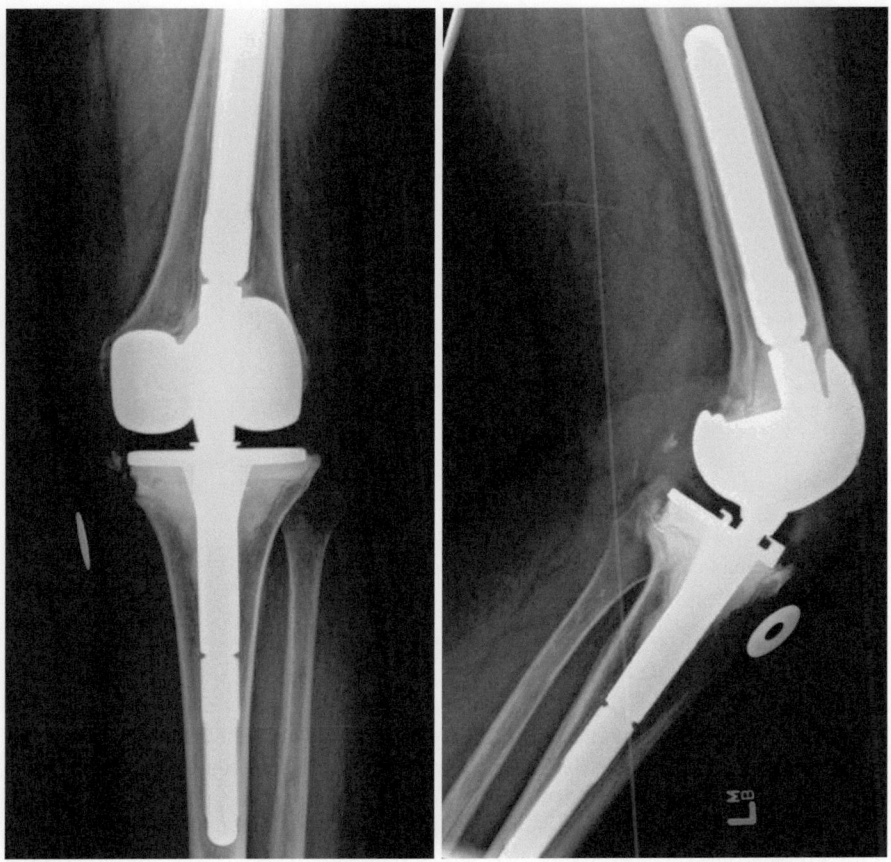

Fig. 1 Radiograph of a 79-year-old male with patellectomy for open patellar fracture and history of uncontrolled diabetes, smoking and poor soft tissue envelope over the knee. This hinge prosthesis was inserted during aseptic revision for ligamentous instability

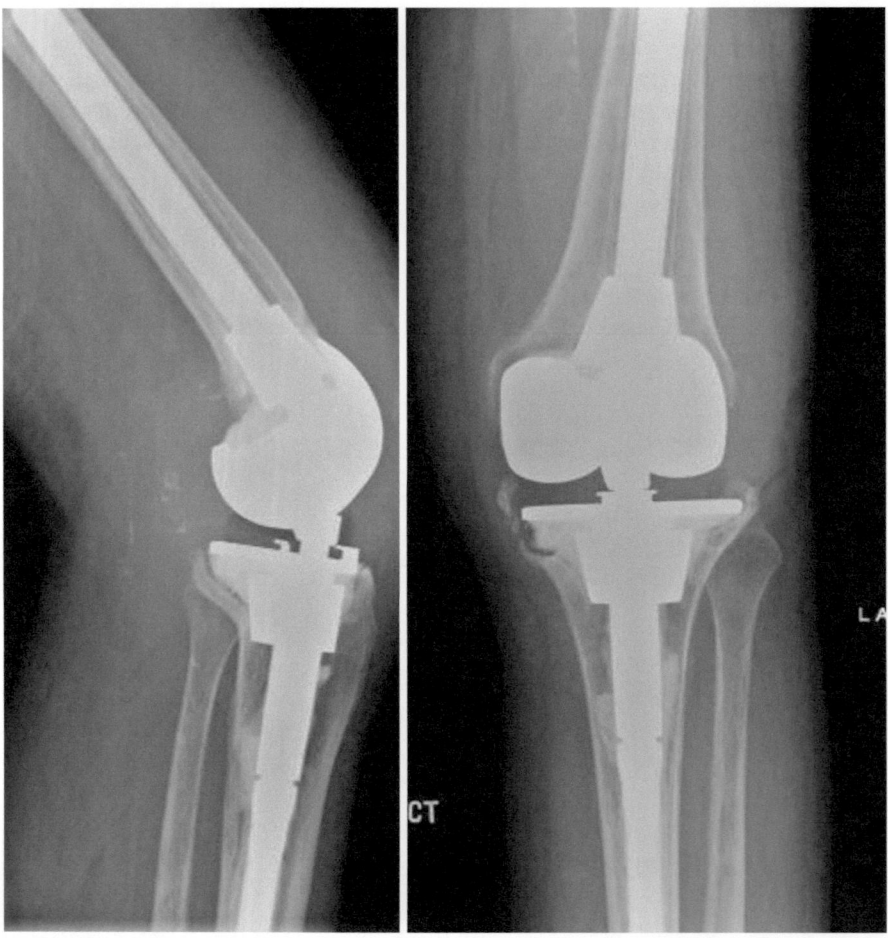

Fig. 2 The patient underwent single-stage revision for PJI management with cones, long hybrid stems, and antibiotic cement. They then developed a polymicrobial and fungal infection. The patient had two DAIR procedures after the single-stage exchange

Repeat One-Stage Revision

Literature reporting on repeat one-stage exchange revision, especially in the hip, has shown to be promising with the added benefit of reducing the number of procedures in half, thereby limited the morbidity incurred by the patient.

Infection-related failure of a septic one-stage exchange revision may be managed with a repeat one-stage exchange. Recent evidence by Neufeld et al. reports on the success rates of repeat septic revision after a one-stage exchange for PJI in revision TKA using a hinge design and fully cemented stems with antibiotic impregnated cement directed by the causative microorganism [7]. Although this cohort included four two-stage exchanges in the re-revision cohort, the majority ($n = 29$) were repeat one-stage exchanges after the initial one-stage exchange for PJI. The 5-year infection-free survival for repeat 1-stage exchange was 59% and the 5-year all-cause survival was 47%. These less than desirable outcomes are similar to those reporting on repeat two-stage revision after a failed 2-stage exchange.

A similar retrospective study from the same institution also reported on the success rates of a repeat one-stage exchange after an initial one-stage exchange for PJI after total hip replacement [8]. The repeat one-stage exchange results in the rTHA cohort were substantially better than those reported for the rTKA cohort. At a mean follow-up of 5.3 years, the results for a total of 32 repeat 1-stage exchange rTHAs were reported. The 5-year infection-free survival rate was 81% and the 5-year all-cause survival rate was 74%.

Based on these findings, the role of repeat 1-stage exchange rTHA appears to deliver more successful outcomes both for infection recurrence and all-cause revision when compared to repeat 1-stage exchange rTKA for recurrent PJI. The reason for the differing success rates in the hip and knee is not fully understood to date but may be related to the increased incidence of PJI in knee arthroplasty over hip arthroplasty in general. Global registries have consistently reported higher rates of periprosthetic joint infection in primary and revision total knee arthroplasty when compared with total hip arthroplasty [9, 10]. This may explain the higher rates of successful infection eradication when repeat single-stage exchange is performed for recurrent hip PJI when compared to recurrent knee PJI.

It is important to note that the literature on repeat one-stage exchange is limited and this should only be attempted in specialty centers with established multidisciplinary teams and expertise in one-stage exchange.

One has to keep in mind that a one-stage exchange may not be possible, especially when long-stem implants are used. In such cases, it is highly likely that the proximal femur will be sufficiently damaged that a proximal femoral replacement may be required.

Two-Stage Revision

Most international arthroplasty units would advocate for a two-stage exchange approach for patients with reinfection after a failed one-stage exchange. Repeat one-stage revisions are not always appropriate or effective, especially in the multiple revision setting for PJI. Slullitel et al. reported the risk factors for failure of a single-stage revision THA performed to treat PJI [11]. In this cohort, the cumulative incidence of septic failure was 19.7% at 5–10 years. Femoral bone loss and obesity were significantly associated with septic failure. The incidence of aseptic failure at 10 years was 12%, where the strongest predictor of aseptic failure was a previous revision to treat PJI. Therefore, we can conclude that the use of a single-stage exchange revision to treat recurrent PJI is likely to fail again due to aseptic causes, even if it remains infection free. For this reason, strong consideration should be given to performing a two-stage revision procedure for recurrence of PJI.

The exact success rate of a two-stage procedure after a single-stage exchange is not widely reported. Neufeld et al. reported on four cases where a septic failure of a single-stage knee exchange was followed by a two-stage revision [7]. The results of these four cases were suboptimal with a 50% revision rate for infection-related failure and one of the four cases requiring an aseptic revision for hinge failure. There have been reports of the comparative success rates of two-stage versus single-stage revision for PJI showing that on multi-variate analysis, a one-stage procedure has a significantly higher adjusted Hazard ratio (HR) for re-revision of 1.72 (95% CI 1.28–2.32) ($p < 0.001$) [12]. This was a sample of 533 patients that all underwent prosthesis removal for PJI management either as a single-stage or two-stage revision thereby supporting the role of two-stage revision over single-stage exchange in the management of PJI. Figures 3, 4 and 5 demonstrate a successful outcome with two-stage revision TKA after a failed single-stage revision.

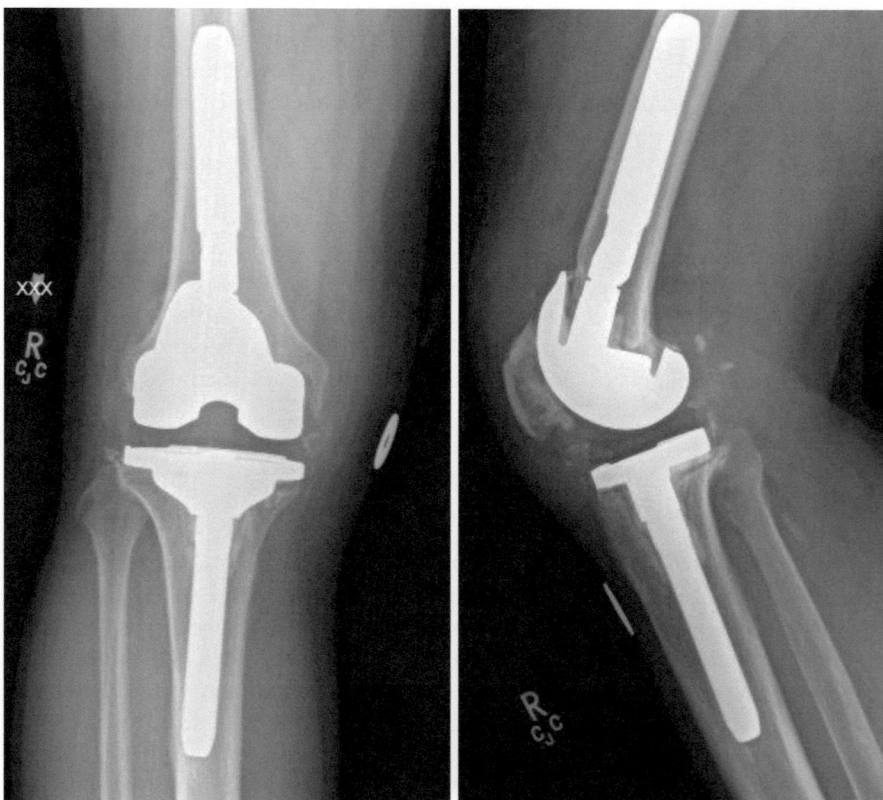

Fig. 3 Knee radiograph of a 66-year-old male post-single-stage exchange for PJI with the use of hybrid stems. Eight months after implantation, failure due to reinfection was reported and peptostreptococcus was grown

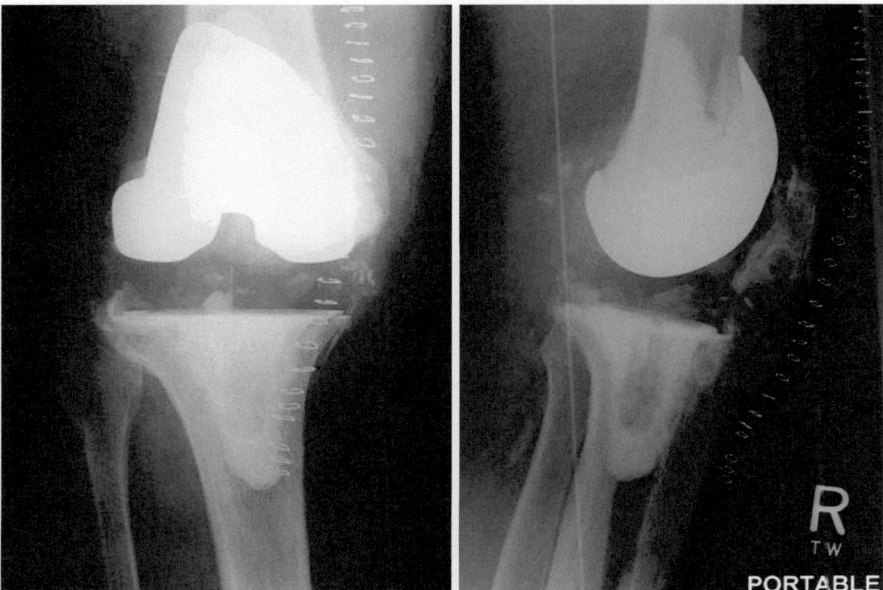

Fig. 4 In this setting, a two-stage revision was deemed to be the best management option and so a cement spacer was inserted for this case

Two-stage revision for PJI is not without risk. The morbidity of hardware removal can be significant in terms of the length of procedure, bone loss, and risk of periprosthetic fracture complicating any further surgery that may be required. Recent evidence by Barry et al. reported on 87 revision TKAs indicated for PJI with extensive hardware already in situ [4]. Extensive instrumentation was defined as ≥ 1 of the following: metaphyseal cones/sleeves, distal femoral replacement, periprosthetic fracture instrumentation, or fully cemented stems measuring >75 mm. Fifty-six were managed with incision and drainage whereas 31 were managed with initiation of 2-stage exchange. Infection eradication was achieved in 62.5% of the DAIR group compared to 67.7% in the two-stage group ($p = 0.62$). In the two-stage group only 41.9% underwent reimplantation with a revision prosthesis and did not require any further surgery or infection, compared to the DAIR group where 62.5% were successfully managed without the need for further surgery to treat infection. The DAIR group also had significantly better function at a mean follow-up of 3.2 years. Ambulation was achieved in 76.8% of the DAIR group compared to 54.8% of the two-stage group ($p = 0.05$). A functional bending knee joint was also more common in the DAIR group (85.7% vs. 45.2%, $p < 0.001$). These impressive results support a more reserved surgical approach to PJI in the presence of extensive metalwork in place of the traditional two-stage approach. Indeed, in this setting, the role of standard 2-stage revision may need to be re-thought entirely.

Fig. 5 Six weeks antibiotic coverage was followed by 6 weeks without antibiotics. Final implantation of components, with the use of press-fit metaphyseal cones, was performed and the patient is known to be infection-free and functioning well at 2 years after most recent surgery

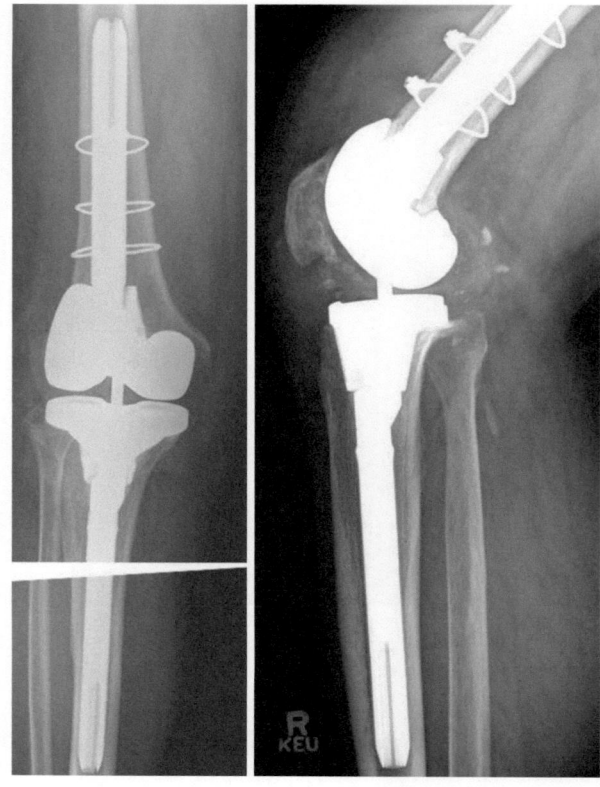

Chronic Antibiotic Suppression

Reinfection rates after one-stage arthroplasty can be as high as 47% with reports commonly observing reinfection within 2 years following the surgical procedure [2, 13, 14]. The failure following one-stage exchange arthroplasty is often associated with an increasing number of virulent bacteria with different isolated pathogens from the initial revision surgery in the 57% of the cases [2, 14].

There is no current general consensus regarding the ideal duration and selection of antibiotic therapy following one-stage arthroplasty surgery [1]. The antibiotic therapy should be selected according to the antibiotic susceptibility of the pathogen isolated, allergies, kidney function, and tolerance to the potential side effects of the drug(s) [15]. Antibiotic treatment should be guided by an infectious disease specialist team with extensive experience in treating PJI.

In the setting of microbiologically-confirmed PJI, extended courses of antimicrobials (12 weeks versus 6 weeks) have been shown in recent literature to afford some benefit in relation to failure secondary to reinfection and should therefore be considered as a standard approach to the revision THA or TKA after a failed one-stage exchange procedure [16, 17]. Fortunately, postoperative courses of antimicrobials need not extend the length of in-hospital stay especially if the isolated pathogen is sensitive to an antimicrobial that has particularly good bioavailability [18].

To date, concerns remain with regard to possible adverse events following chronic suppression antibiotic therapy such as rash and gastro-intestinal intolerance but the development of multi-resistant pathogens is the most concerning sequela [4]. It should be noted that if patients remain infection-free after 5 years from the revision surgery, infection is unlikely to recur at longer follow-up [11]. Reinfection after one-stage exchange arthroplasty can be a major challenge, particularly when concerning immunocompromised patients [19]. Ji et al. reviewed 17 patients, who underwent one-stage revision and nine of them had recurrence of infections. Seven of the nine failures were treated with chronic suppressive antibiotic therapy. They also found a higher incidence of fungal PJI, which is generally considered to be more difficult to eradicate than bacterial infections. Chronic suppressive antibiotic therapy consisted of levofloxacin and rifampicin therapy in bacterial infections, whereas fluconazole was added in fungal cases.

Another challenge is the treatment of Enterococcal infections, which occurs in 2–7% of PJI in the knee and hip joints. Rossmann et al. found an infection recurrence rate of 37.5% following one-stage knee exchange arthroplasty with a 60% rate of non-enterococcal infections after a mean time of 22 months [20]. These infections are rare and often have polymicrobial association where a reliable treatment algorithm has not yet been developed. Similarly, Renz et al. found that 17% of the patients had a new episode of PJI at a later stage caused by a different pathogen than Enterococcus [21].

On the contrary, Neufeld et al. retrospectively reviewed a total of 29 septic repeated one-stage revision total knee arthroplasties which were undertaken after a failed one-stage exchange [7]. Only three patients continued taking antibiotics up to 6 months due to streptococcal infection; however, no patients required chronic antibiotic suppression. Further high-powered, high-quality prospective randomized controlled studies are required to inform future algorithms and protocols in this area. Of note, the study by Bernard et al. did not include repeat one-stage exchange procedures and so this is still an area that needs to be more rigorously investigated in the future [16]. However, considering the high stakes with failure after a repeat revision after septic failure of one-stage exchange, prolonged suppressive antibiotics, even for life if tolerated, would be recommended especially in high risk patients.

Arthrodesis

Arthrodesis is considered to be a viable option in failed one-stage arthroplasty to reduce the patient's pain, reduce the likelihood of further revision, and provide a stable joint for mobilization. Citak et al. reviewed 93 patients who underwent subsequent revision following one-stage revision knee arthroplasty [2]. Five of them (6%) underwent arthrodesis. Similarly, Rossmann et al. reported that 1 of 40 patients (3%) required a permanent arthrodesis after one-stage revision knee arthroplasty [20].

Arthrodesis in the presence of reinfection may lead to an infected non-union at the fusion site. If unable to achieve a stable joint fusion to facilitate mobilization, amputation may be required to create a stump that can be used for socket fitting. A transcutaneous osseointegration prosthesis can only be used if there is absolutely no evidence of recurrent or residual infection.

Resection Arthroplasty, Amputation, and Osseointegration

Numerous salvage options are available for the surgical management of end-stage recurrent PJI. Resection arthroplasty is a viable option with relatively low morbidity. It may be performed as an intentionally definitive procedure or it may be performed as the first of a planned two-stage procedure where reimplantation never actually comes to fruition for a number of reasons [22]. Significant medical comorbidities and resistant infections are risks for never reimplanting a joint after resection arthroplasty.

Above-knee amputation is a salvage procedure that may be performed after revision one-stage arthroplasty fails to eradicate PJI. Citak et al. [2] reviewed 93 patients, who underwent subsequent revision following one-stage revision knee arthroplasty. Two of them (2%) required amputation of the affected limb. Rossmann et al. reported that two patients (5%) required above-knee amputations after their revision procedure to treat a polymicrobial enterococcal PJI and subsequent reinfection [17]. Amputation is the end-stage surgical option for a failed single-stage revision for PJI.

Transfemoral amputations pose a greater limitation to patient function with increasing energy requirements to mobilize. In this setting, function may be significantly improved through the use of a transcutaneous osseointegration (OI) device which realigns the bony skeleton along its mechanical axis, provides proprioception to the lower limb, and avoids all the issues with conventional socket use. Although in their infancy, OI devices have been shown to greatly improve the functioning of amputee patients undergoing this procedure [23]. Interestingly, specifically in the setting of amputation following TKA PJI, there is a small series reporting that transfemoral osseointegration has been shown to confer significantly better mobility and quality of life when compared to knee fusion or transfemoral amputation with traditional socket prostheses following an infected TKR in the short term [24]. The high rate of OI reintervention is an issue that will be targeted in future innovation and research so that patient function after amputation may be significantly improved. Currently, patients with traumatic amputations seem to have the best outcomes following OI and the PJI literature is significantly more limited. Although unknown, the PJI amputation patient population is likely to have a higher reinfection and failure rate with OI as well.

Conclusion

Reinfection after a one-stage exchange revision for PJI is a devastating complication with significant morbidity associated and there is a paucity of literature in this patient population. Similar to the literature on patients undergoing a repeat two-stage exchange after a failed two-stage exchange for PJI, patients with a reinfection after a one-stage exchange should be counseled on the high rates of infection-related failure and re-revision. Although not widely published, the body of evidence available supports the use of DAIR procedures, particularly in the context of extensive hardware. Repeat one-stage revision may be a reasonable option but is more likely to successfully eradicate PJI in the hip rather than the knee. A repeat one-stage revision should only be attempted in specialized centers and most centers would advocate for a repeat two-stage revision for this patient population. However, the superiority of a two-stage compared to a one-stage revision in this patient population is unknown.

Resection arthroplasty, arthrodesis, and amputation are salvage options and transcutaneous osseointegration surgery may significantly improve the functional outcomes of patients who have already undergone amputation in this setting. Chronic antimicrobial suppression is a non-invasive option with well documented repercussions including the emergence of antimicrobial resistance.

As with all surgical complications, prevention is preferable to treatment. Therefore, the risk factors mentioned at the beginning of this chapter that are known to increase the failure of single-stage exchange should be carefully observed and optimized prior to surgery.

References

1. Abdelaziz H, Grüber H, Gehrke T, Salber J, Citak M. What are the factors associated with re-revision after one-stage revision for periprosthetic joint infection of the hip? A case-control study. Clin Orthop Relat Res. 2019;477(10):2258–63. https://doi.org/10.1097/CORR.0000000000000780.
2. Citak M, Friedenstab J, Abdelaziz H, et al. Risk factors for failure after 1-stage exchange total knee arthroplasty in the management of periprosthetic joint infection. J Bone Joint Surg Am. 2019;101(12):1061–9. https://doi.org/10.2106/JBJS.18.00947.
3. Abdelaziz H, Schröder M, Shum Tien C, et al. Resection of the proximal femur during one-stage revision for infected hip arthroplasty : risk factors and effectiveness. Bone Joint J. 2021;103-B(11):1678–85. https://doi.org/10.1302/0301-620X.103B11.BJJ-2021-0022.R1.
4. Barry JJ, Geary MB, Riesgo AM, Odum SM, Fehring TK, Springer BD. Irrigation and debridement with chronic antibiotic suppression is as effective as 2-stage exchange in revision Total knee arthroplasty with extensive instrumentation. J Bone Joint Surg Am. 2021;103(1):53–63. https://doi.org/10.2106/JBJS.20.00240.
5. Vahedi H, Aali-Rezaie A, Shahi A, Conway JD. Irrigation, Débridement, and implant retention for recurrence of Periprosthetic joint infection following two-stage revision Total knee arthroplasty: a matched cohort study. J Arthroplast. 2019;34(8):1772–5. https://doi.org/10.1016/j.arth.2019.04.009.
6. Veerman K, Raessens J, Telgt D, Smulders K, Goosen JHM. Debridement, antibiotics, and implant retention after revision arthroplasty: antibiotic mismatch, timing, and repeated DAIR associated with poor outcome. Bone Joint J. 2022;104-B(4):464–71. https://doi.org/10.1302/0301-620X.104B4.BJJ-2021-1264.R1.
7. Neufeld ME, Liechti EF, Soto F, et al. High revision rates following repeat septic revision after failed one-stage exchange for periprosthetic joint infection in total knee arthroplasty. Bone Joint J. 2022;104-B(3):386–93. https://doi.org/10.1302/0301-620X.104B3.BJJ-2021-0481.R2.
8. Liechti EF, Neufeld ME, Soto F, et al. Favourable outcomes of repeat one-stage exchange for periprosthetic joint infection of the hip. Bone Joint J. 2022;104-B(1):27–33. https://doi.org/10.1302/0301-620X.104B1.BJJ-2021-0970.R1.
9. Huotari K, Peltola M, Jämsen E. The incidence of late prosthetic joint infections: a registry-based study of 112,708 primary hip and knee replacements. Acta Orthop. 2015;86(3):321–5. https://doi.org/10.3109/17453674.2015.1035173.

10. https://reports.njrcentre.org.uk/Portals/0/PDFdownloads/NJR%2018th%20Annual%20 Report%202021.pdf.
11. Slullitel PA, Oñativia JI, Zanotti G, Comba F, Piccaluga F, Buttaro MA. One-stage exchange should be avoided in periprosthetic joint infection cases with massive femoral bone loss or with history of any failed revision to treat periprosthetic joint infection. Bone Joint J. 2021;103-B(7):1247–53. https://doi.org/10.1302/0301-620X.103B7.BJJ-2020-2155.R1.
12. Kandel CE, Jenkinson R, Daneman N, et al. Predictors of treatment failure for hip and knee prosthetic joint infections in the setting of 1-and 2-stage exchange arthroplasty: a multicenter retrospective cohort. Open Forum Infect Dis. 2019;6(11):ofz452. Published 2019 Oct 21. https://doi.org/10.1093/ofid/ofz452.
13. Masters JP, Smith NA, Foguet P, Reed M, Parsons H, Sprowson AP. A systematic review of the evidence for single stage and two stage revision of infected knee replacement. BMC Musculoskelet Disord. 2013;14:222.
14. Akkaya M, Vles G, Bakhtiari IG, Sandiford A, Salber J, Gehrke T, Citak M. What is the rate of reinfection with different and difficult-to-treat bacteria after failed one-stage septic knee exchange? Int Orthop. 2022;46(4):687–95.
15. Myers TG, Lipof JS, Chen AF, Ricciardi BF. Antibiotic stewardship for total joint arthroplasty in 2020. J Am Acad Orthop Surg. 2020;28:e793–802.
16. Bernard L, Arvieux C, Brunschweiler B, Touchais S, Ansart S, Bru JP, Oziol E, Boeri C, Gras G, Druon J, Rosset P, Senneville E, Bentayeb H, Bouhour D, Le Moal G, Michon J, Aumaître H, Forestier E, Laffosse JM, Begué T, Chirouze C, Dauchy FA, Devaud E, Martha B, Burgot D, Boutoille D, Stindel E, Dinh A, Bemer P, Giraudeau B, Issartel B, Caille A. Antibiotic therapy for 6 or 12 weeks for prosthetic joint infection. N Engl J Med. 2021;384(21):1991–2001. https://doi.org/10.1056/NEJMoa2020198. PMID: 34042388.
17. Frank JM, Kayupov E, Moric M, Segreti J, Hansen E, Hartman C, Okroj K, Belden K, Roslund B, Silibovsky R, Parvizi J, Della Valle CJ, Knee Society Research Group. The Mark Coventry, MD. Award: oral antibiotics reduce reinfection after two-stage exchange: a multicenter, randomized controlled trial. Clin Orthop Relat Res. 2017;475(1):56–61. https://doi.org/10.1007/s11999-016-4890-4. PMID: 27387759; PMCID: PMC5174034.
18. Li HK, Rombach I, Zambellas R, Walker AS, McNally MA, Atkins BL, Lipsky BA, Hughes HC, Bose D, Kümin M, Scarborough C, Matthews PC, Brent AJ, Lomas J, Gundle R, Rogers M, Taylor A, Angus B, Byren I, Berendt AR, Warren S, Fitzgerald FE, Mack DJF, Hopkins S, Folb J, Reynolds HE, Moore E, Marshall J, Jenkins N, Moran CE, Woodhouse AF, Stafford S, Seaton RA, Vallance C, Hemsley CJ, Bisnauthsing K, Sandoe JAT, Aggarwal I, Ellis SC, Bunn DJ, Sutherland RK, Barlow G, Cooper C, Geue C, McMeekin N, Briggs AH, Sendi P, Khatamzas E, Wangrangsimakul T, Wong THN, Barrett LK, Alvand A, Old CF, Bostock J, Paul J, Cooke G, Thwaites GE, Bejon P, Scarborough M, OVIVA Trial Collaborators. Oral versus intravenous antibiotics for bone and joint infection. N Engl J Med. 2019;380(5):425–36. https://doi.org/10.1056/NEJMoa1710926. PMID: 30699315; PMCID: PMC6522347.
19. Ji B, Zhang X, Xu B, et al. The fate of immunocompromised patients in the treatment of chronic periprosthetic joint infection: a single-centre experience. Int Orthopaedics (SICOT). 2018;42:487–98.
20. Rossmann M, Minde T, Citak M, Gehrke T, Sandiford NA, Klatte TO, Abdelaziz H. High rate of reinfection with new bacteria following one-stage exchange for Enterococcal Periprosthetic infection of the knee: a single-center study. J Arthroplast. 2021;36(2):711–6.
21. Renz N, Trebse R, Akgün D, Perka C, Trampuz A. Enterococcal periprosthetic joint infection: clinical and microbiological findings from an 8-year retro-spective cohort study. BMC Infect Dis. 2019;19:1083.
22. Lin YH, Chang CJ, Chang CW, Chen YC, Tai TW. The reasons for and mortality of patients unable to receive reimplantation after resection arthroplasty for chronic hip periprosthetic infection. Int Orthop. 2022;46(3):465–72. https://doi.org/10.1007/s00264-021-05254-4. Epub 2021 Nov 8. Erratum in: Int Orthop. 2022 Jan 19;: PMID: 34746981.

23. Reif TJ, Khabyeh-Hasbani N, Jaime KM, Sheridan GA, Otterburn DM, Rozbruch SR. Early experience with femoral and tibial bone-anchored osseointegration prostheses. JB JS Open Access. 2021;6(3):e21.00072. Published 2021 Sep 3. https://doi.org/10.2106/JBJS.OA.21.00072.
24. Akhtar MA, Hoellwarth JS, Tetsworth K, Oomatia A, Al MM. Osseointegration following Transfemoral amputation after infected Total knee replacement: a case series of 10 patients with a mean follow-up of 5 years. Arthroplast Today. 2022;16:21–30. Published 2022 May 21. https://doi.org/10.1016/j.artd.2022.04.008.

Knee Arthrodesis: Salvage Procedure After Failed Total Knee Arthroplasty

Dhanasekara Raja Palanisami,
Raja Bhaskara Rajasekaran,
Soundarrajan Dhanasekaran, Rithika Singh,
Duncan Whitwell, and Shanmuganathan Rajasekaran

Abbreviations

IMN	Intramedullary Nail
KA	Knee Arthrodesis
PJI	Periprosthetic joint infection
TKA	Total Knee Arthroplasty

Although the surgeon may consider an arthrodesis of the knee to be a poor outcome, a limb with a fusion is more efficient and functional than is one with an above-the-knee amputation—[1].

Introduction

With the increase in the aging population globally, there has been a proportional increase in total knee arthroplasty (TKA) procedures. Estimates show that by 2030, the number of TKA procedures will grow by more than 650% [2]. Furthermore, the demand for revision TKA following failed primary TKA is expected to grow by nearly 600% in the next 5 years [2–4]. As these numbers grow, there are also increased chances of clinicians needing to manage cases of multiple failed TKAs leading to an un reconstructible TKA [5]. This subset of patients offers significant challenges to the surgeon due to complexities involved with the decreased remaining native bone for revision surgery, poor skin condition, and managing patients'

D. R. Palanisami · R. B. Rajasekaran (✉) · S. Dhanasekaran · R. Singh · S. Rajasekaran
Department of Orthopaedics, Ganga Medical Centre & Hospitals Pvt. Ltd, Coimbatore, India

D. Whitwell
Nuffield Orthopaedic Centre Headington, Oxford, UK
e-mail: duncan.whitwell@ndorms.ox.ac.uk

© The Author(s), under exclusive license to Springer Nature
Switzerland AG 2024
M. Citak et al. (eds.), *One-Stage Septic Revision Arthroplasty*,
https://doi.org/10.1007/978-3-031-59160-0_10

expectations after the procedure. In these circumstances, knee arthrodesis (KA) can be a useful salvage option in restoring the weight-bearing ability of the patient, in addition to providing a stable extremity. The cumulative incidence of KA following failed TKA due to periprosthetic joint infection (PJI) is 0.26%, as per one reported study [6]. Clinicians need to be convinced regarding the benefit of KA, compared to other treatment options, including transfemoral amputations and above-knee amputations.

In this chapter, we will discuss the indications, principles, and techniques for knee arthrodesis after the failure of TKA due to recurrent PJI.

Indications and Contraindications of Knee Arthrodesis After Failed TKA

A failed TKA, which is unreconstructible, is a good option for knee arthrodesis. The various indications and contraindications have been listed in Table 1. Disrupted extensor mechanisms which are very challenging to reconstruct, large bone defects around the knee, poor soft-tissue coverage, and painful knee with arthrofibrosis are indications that may warrant KA [1, 5]. However, the most standard indication for KA after failed TKA is recurrent PJI.

The contraindications to KA include prior contralateral KA, ipsilateral hip arthrodesis or a contralateral transfemoral amputation [5, 6]. These associated conditions would significantly impact the compensatory mechanisms during the gait cycle, thereby markedly increasing energy expenditure. Studies have shown that oxygen consumption is roughly 30% higher when walking with a KA than normal walking [7–9]. KA is shown to increase the stress transfer across the ipsilateral knee and hip, so proper examination of these joints to assess their mobility is essential before considering KA [5]. Degenerative lumbar spine disease is also a relative contraindication, as compensatory forces can worsen the degeneration after KA [10].

Table 1 Key points involved in decision-making while performing knee arthrodesis

Indications	Contraindications
– Recurrent PJI	– Contralateral knee arthrodesis
– Large bone defects	– Ipsilateral hip arthrodesis
– Disrupted extensor mechanism, which is not reconstructible	– Transfemoral amputation
– Poor soft-tissue cover	– Degenerative lumbar spine disease (relative contraindication)
– Painful knee with severe arthrofibrosis	

When to Do A Knee Arthrodesis After Failed TKA?

The timing to do a KA has always been debated. Coupled with the choice of surgery, it is a dilemma for surgeons to decide on KA for a failed TKA after PJI. KA is often considered as an unfavorable option by surgeons and hence is only preferred as a last resort after failed TKA. However, by this time, due to the multiple revision surgeries, there is significant bone loss thereby jeopardizing the fusion procedure [5, 11]. KA performed after multiple revisions have poor outcomes due to poor bone stock available to achieve union [12]. Hence, timing of surgery is crucial, to achieve optimal outcomes with KA.

Repeat surgical intervention after a failed 2-stage revision for PJI is associated with poorer outcomes. Infection control in a repeat 2-stage revision procedure failed in 38.4% of patients [13]. Hence, it is recommended that KA be considered after one failed two-stage revision surgery to achieve favorable outcomes. Adequate counseling after a failed infected TKA is essential to manage patient expectations, when the surgeon is considering KA.

Principles of Knee Arthrodesis

The key principles for KA after PJI revolve around the following factors: adequate infection control, host optimization, optimal knee fusion position, achieving maximum bone-to-bone contact at the site of fusion, and achieving adequate limb length. Gaining adequate control of modifiable risk factors influencing wound healing, primarily diabetes should be addressed appropriately before surgery. Involving multiple clinical teams, especially an infectious disease specialist or an Infection multidisciplinary team, has proven beneficial [14, 15]. Usually revision surgeries around the knee are associated with poor skin condition, necessitating plastic surgery inputs for adequate soft-tissue coverage. Acute shortening during KA may result in skin-closure during surgery.

Usually 10–15° of flexion at the knee joint is recommended, as it assists with sitting and also improves gait speed [1]. Keeping the limb about 1.5 cm shorter than the contralateral limb is advisable, as it allows easier clearance from the ground during walking. Five to seven degree of valgus is advisable on the coronal plane, to decrease varus stress on the hip and ankle joint [16]. Surgical planning needs to be done to achieve maximum bone contact at the fusion site, to achieve union. Often the question of preserving the extensor mechanism in cases of knee fusion remains. Still, it is advisable to keep it wherever possible, as it would lead to excessive strain on the psoas while walking. A shoe raise can easily manage up to 5 cm of limb shortening.

Commonly used modalities for KA include compression plating, external fixator, and intramedullary nailing (IMN). Each modality has specific advantages, and clinicians will need to tailor their method of KA, based on the availability of expertise, and also the clinical condition of the patient.

Compression Plating

Compression plating is a commonly employed procedure with a good outcome in the hands of the authors. One of this procedure's main prerequisites is having adequate bone available for fusion. The advantage is that a rigid fixation can be achieved. Published reports show an excellent union rate in their respective series [17, 18]. The authors also reported that 18% of their patients developed femoral stress fractures. Staggering of the locking plates may prevent this late complication. Another disadvantage of this procedure is that, post-surgery, immediate weight-bearing cannot be initiated as compared to other treatment modalities. In our practice, we prefer to use dual plates in cases with minimal bone loss (Fig. 1) and prefer to place each plate in a different plane.

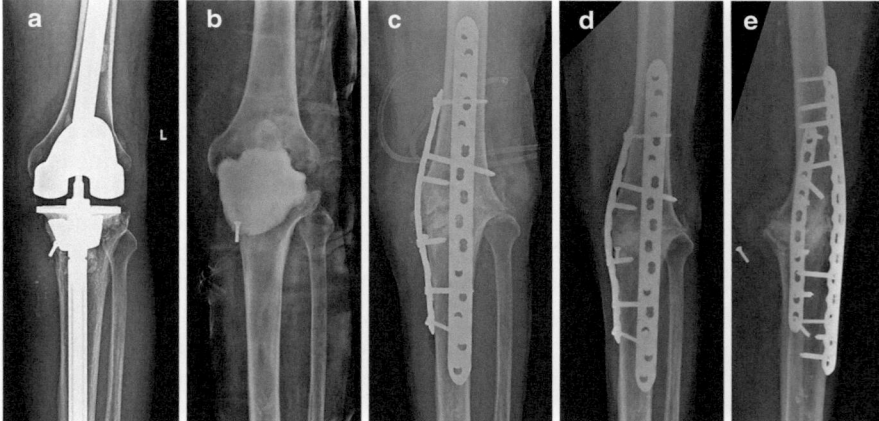

Fig. 1 Persistent gram-negative PJI after two attempts at DAIR (debridement, antibiotics, and implant retention) (**a**), was managed with prosthesis removal and cement spacer application (**b**) at first stage. After infection control, knee arthrodesis with locking plates was done after shortening and achieving adequate compression at bony ends (**c**). At 2-year follow-up (**d, e**), a complete union is seen with a limb shortening of 2 cm, managed with shoe raise

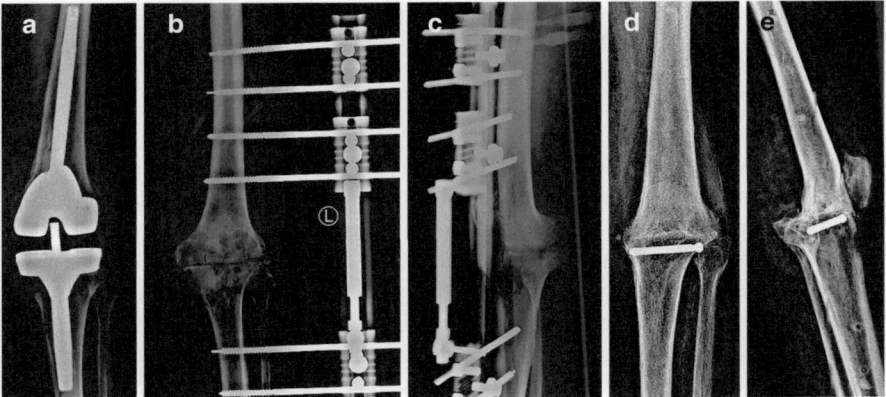

Fig. 2 One-stage KA: Failed TKA with persistent infection (**a**) managed with KA (**b, c**) using uniplanar external fixator with adequate bone contact at the fusion site. Fusion was seen at 6 months, infection was controlled, after which the fixator was removed (**d, e**)

External Fixators

External fixator devices can be performed through small incisions and in case of fulminant infections. Compression using external fixators can be performed as a uniplanar construct (Fig. 2), or biplanar construct, and in some cases, a circular construct. Circular constructs offer excellent stability and are also advantageous as simultaneous lengthening in the femur or tibia (distraction osteogenesis) can be done, while compressing the union site [19]. In cases with massive bone loss, external fixators are useful as acute shortening to achieve union may not be possible. Gradual lengthening can be done in such cases. On the downside, external fixators have an increased rate of pin-tract infections, increased chances of neurovascular injuries, and stress fractures through pin-tracts. Care must be taken to remove the pins, only after radiological evidence of bony union at the fusion site, as there is an increased preponderance to refracture after frame removal [20]. In such cases, using an IMN or plate after fusion is advisable. Modern hexapod frames offer advantages where the surgeon can tailor the construct to achieve the desired alignment [21].

Intramedullary Nails (IMN)

The knowledge of a familiar technique of nailing for most surgeons makes it a preferred method for managing KA among many surgeons. Following debridement at the fusion site, long IMNs are inserted through the piriformis fossa (antegrade approach) spanning the knee joint up to the desired level at the tibia. Locking bolts are used proximally and distally [5]. Nowadays, newer systems with increased modularity have also been introduced, which allow surgeons to pass the nail through the knee incision [22]. The TITAN (KAM) arthrodesis system is a modular arthrodesis IMN, providing a cementless stem for diaphyseal anchorage. Cementless modular systems have shown promising results with regard to prosthesis survivorship, limb length discrepancy, and functional outcome [22, 23]. Even in the hands of the authors, these systems provide robust fixation and also can be employed in cases with significant bone loss. Surgeons have also advocated silver-coated IMNs in cases of persistent infection, showing favorable results [23, 24]. In an unpublished series of seven cases using IMN arthrodesis system from the authors institution, six patients had good outcomes at their final follow-up. Two patients, who had minimal bone gap at the fusion site, also showed union at an average of 9 months post-surgery (Fig. 3). However, one patient still has persistent infection, and the further treatment is still a dilemma, as removing these nails is very challenging. Cortical bone windows are needed, and apart from jeopardizing the fusion site, further management options are sparse. Hence, removing these stems is very challenging in cases of re-infection or recurrent infection.

In cases of poor soft-tissue coverage and having an ipsilateral hip prosthesis, these systems can be challenging and are not recommended. Recently, antibiotic-coated IMNs have been advocated for controlling infection and achieving fusion in a single stage [5, 20, 25]. Based on the previous culture and sensitivity, antibiotic-coated cement is used in addition to a silicone tube to fabricate the IMN [5].

To minimize the time for fusion, some authors have advocated using a circular frame along with IMN [20]. Combining an IMN with antibiotic cement can assist in the temporary elution of antibiotics against further infection. In cases of active infection, some authors advocate doing a two-stage KA. The use of antibiotic-loaded IMN after debridement as a temporary spacer can be considered in such cases, and after a period of 6–8 weeks, definitive fusion can be done (Fig. 4).

Surgeons can tailor their surgical strategy based on available options while performing KA, aiming to achieve solid fusion, maintaining adequate limb length, and controlling infection (Table 2).

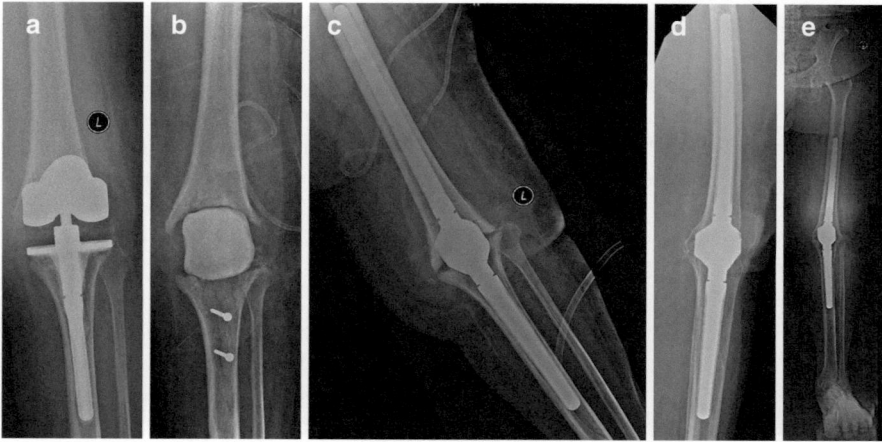

Fig. 3 Failed TKA due to PJI (**a, b**) was managed with prosthesis removal and cement spacer application after tibial tubercle osteotomy at first stage. Later, a modular KAM-TITAN IMN system was used to achieve fusion (**c**). Note the fusion of the bony edges (**d, e**) at 1 year post-surgery

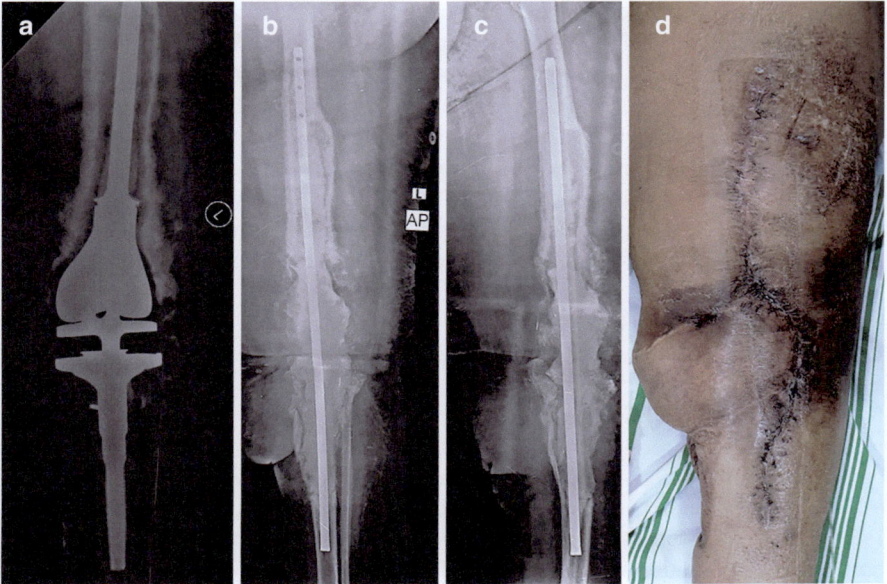

Fig. 4 Six attempts at infection eradication in a primary TKA presented with fulminant infection and discharging pus with septic loosening of endoprosthesis (**a**) in a 54-year old female. Thorough debridement, removal of the prosthesis, and K-nail with antibiotic-loaded cement was inserted as a temporary spacer to control infection (**b, c**). Note the skin flap done to achieve soft-tissue cover (**d**). Once adequate infection control is achieved, permanent KA can be considered using IMN prosthesis

Table 2 Tips in decision-making and surgical planning to achieve favorable outcomes in knee arthrodesis (KA) following failed TKA

– Combining the opinion of a microbiologist and a plastic surgeon is beneficial to manage antibiotics in infection and wound coverage, respectively
– Minimal shortening (about 1.5 cm) compared to the contralateral limb is advised, as it helps with lift-off while walking
– Achieving solid fusion, maintaining limb length, and preventing recurrent infection must be the goals aimed at while planning KA after failed TKA
– KA can be considered after one failed attempt at two-stage revision TKA to have adequate bone stock to achieve fusion
– The use of IMN has shown increased union rates compared to other modalities
– In cases of active infection, antibiotic cement-loaded IMN with interlocking bolts can be considered as a single-stage intervention

One-Stage Knee Arthrodesis After Failed TKA

As discussed earlier, KA after failed TKA can be performed either as a one-stage or two-stage procedure. The presence of active infection is one of the significant determinants of decision-making. In cases of stiff knees or knees with deficient extensor mechanisms, in the absence of infection, one-stage KA is the norm. Even in cases of infection, thorough debridement, removal of components, and KA can be done. In a study involving 27 patients with one-stage KA for infected PJI, the authors reported the persistence of infection in 14.8% of patients [26]. More interestingly, all patients in their series, including the single patient who underwent amputation, indicated choosing arthrodesis again, showing the procedure's efficacy over amputation. While the principles and techniques regarding KA remain the same, decision-making is essential, and the role of a multidisciplinary team is beneficial in collective decision-making when planning for 1-stage KA. In active infection, eternal fixation devices, can be used as a viable option to achieve fusion (Fig. 2).

Conclusion

KA following failed TKA, especially an infected TKA is a viable option and can provide a stable extremity. Before convincing the patient, the surgeon needs to be confident regarding the benefits of this procedure and its efficacy. While the timing of KA is controversial, it may be considered after one failed attempt at two-stage revision to increase fusion rates. KA provides better functional outcomes than above-knee amputation when managing the failure of infected TKAs. Various techniques are available, and surgeons should utilize them based on available expertise and clinical indications. Use of IMN for arthrodesis results in higher fusion rates. Newer techniques involving antibiotic-impregnated cement spacers to bridge bone defects show promise, but long-te en.

Conflict of Interest The authors declare no conflict of interest.

References

1. Conway JD, Mont MA, Bezwada HP. Arthrodesis of the knee. J Bone Joint Surg Am. 2004;86(4):835–48. https://doi.org/10.2106/00004623-200404000-00027.
2. Kurtz S, Ong K, Lau E, Mowat F, Halpern M. Projections of primary and revision hip and knee arthroplasty in the United States from 2005 to 2030. J Bone Joint Surg Am. 2007;89(4):780–5. https://doi.org/10.2106/JBJS.F.00222.
3. Brown ML, Javidan P, Early S, Bugbee W. Evolving etiologies and rates of revision total knee arthroplasty: a 10-year institutional report. Arthroplasty. 2022;4(1):39. https://doi.org/10.1186/s42836-022-00134-7. PMID: 36008846. PMCID: PMC9404596.
4. Sabah SA, von Fritsch L, Khan T, Shearman AD, Rajasekaran RB, Oxford Revision Arthroplasty Group, Beard DJ, Price AJ, Alvand A. Revision total knee replacement case-mix at a major revision centre. J Exp Orthop. 2022;9(1):34. https://doi.org/10.1186/s40634-022-00462-2. PMID: 35422112; PMCID: PMC9010489.
5. Makhdom AM, Fragomen A, Rozbruch SR. Knee arthrodesis after failed total knee arthroplasty. J Bone Joint Surg Am. 2019;101(7):650–60. https://doi.org/10.2106/JBJS.18.00191.
6. Gottfriedsen TB, Schrøder HM, Odgaard A. Knee arthrodesis after failure of knee arthroplasty: a Nationwide register-based study. J Bone Joint Surg Am. 2016;98(16):1370–7. https://doi.org/10.2106/JBJS.15.01363.
7. Datta D, Heller B, Howitt J. A comparative evaluation of oxygen consumption and gait pattern in amputees using intelligent prostheses and conventionally damped knee swing-phase control. Clin Rehabil. 2005;19(4):398–403. https://doi.org/10.1191/0269215505cr805oa.

8. Preininger B, Matziolis G, Perka C. Knee arthrodesis. In: Bentley G, editor. European surgical orthopaedics and traumatology. Berlin: Springer; 2014. https://doi.org/10.1007/978-3-642-34746-7_132.
9. Spina M, Gualdrini G, Fosco M, Giunti A. Knee arthrodesis with the Ilizarov external fixator as treatment for septic failure of knee arthroplasty. J Orthop Traumatol. 2010;11(2):81–8. https://doi.org/10.1007/s10195-010-0089-8. Epub 2010 Apr 28. PMID: 20425133; PMCID: PMC2896581.
10. Damron TA, McBeath AA. Arthrodesis following failed total knee arthroplasty: comprehensive review and meta-analysis of recent literature. Orthopedics. 1995;18(4):361–8. https://doi.org/10.3928/0147-7447-19950401-10.
11. Brodersen MP, Fitzgerald RH Jr, Peterson LF, Coventry MB, Bryan RS. Arthrodesis of the knee following failed total knee arthroplasty. J Bone Joint Surg Am. 1979;61(2):181–5.
12. Hak DJ, Lieberman JR, Finerman GA. Single plane and biplane external fixators for knee arthrodesis. Clin Orthop Relat Res. 1995;316:134–44.
13. Kheir MM, Tan TL, Gomez MM, Chen AF, Parvizi J. Patients with failed prior two-stage exchange have poor outcomes after further surgical intervention. J Arthroplast. 2017;32(4):1262–5. https://doi.org/10.1016/j.arth.2016.10.008. Epub 2016 Oct 20.
14. Zahar A, Sarungi M. Diagnosis and management of the infected total knee replacement: a practical surgical guide. J Exp Orthop. 2021;8(1):14. https://doi.org/10.1186/s40634-021-00333-2. PMID: 33619607; PMCID: PMC7900357.
15. Rajasekaran RB, Whitwell D, Cosker TDA, Gibbons CLMH, Carr A. Will virtual multidisciplinary team meetings become the norm for musculoskeletal oncology care following the COVID-19 pandemic?—experience from a tertiary sarcoma Centre. BMC Musculoskelet Disord. 2021;22(1):18. https://doi.org/10.1186/s12891-020-03925-8. PMID: 33402136; PMCID: PMC7784619.
16. Puranen J, Kortelainen P, Jalovaara P. Arthrodesis of the knee with intramedullary nail fixation. J Bone Joint Surg Am. 1990;72(3):433–42.
17. Kuo AC, Meehan JP, Lee M. Knee fusion using dual platings with the locking compression plate. J Arthroplast. 2005;20(6):772–6. https://doi.org/10.1016/j.arth.2005.06.003.
18. Nichols SJ, Landon GC, Tullos HS. Arthrodesis with dual plates after failed total knee arthroplasty. J Bone Joint Surg Am. 1991;73(7):1020–4.
19. Nozaka K, Miyakoshi N, Hongo M, Kasukawa Y, Saito H, Kijima H, Tsuchie H, Mita M, Shimada Y. Effectiveness of circular external fixator in periprosthetic fractures around the knee. BMC Musculoskelet Disord. 2020;21(1):317. https://doi.org/10.1186/s12891-020-03352-9. PMID: 32438922; PMCID: PMC7243335.
20. Kuchinad R, Fourman MS, Fragomen AT, Rozbruch SR. Knee arthrodesis as limb salvage for complex failures of total knee arthroplasty. J Arthroplast. 2014;29(11):2150–5. https://doi.org/10.1016/j.arth.2014.06.021. Epub 2014 Jul 4.
21. Gathen M, Schmolders J, Wimmer MD, Gravius N, Randau TM, Gravius S, Friedrich M. Modulares Kniearthrodesesystem TITAN (KAM-TITAN) nach fehlgeschlagener Knieendoprothetik : operative Technik und klinische Ergebnisse [modular arthrodesis system TITAN (KAM-TITAN) after failed revision total knee arthroplasty : operative technique and clinical experience]. Oper Orthop Traumatol. 2020;32(1):58–72. German. Epub 2019 Jun 26. https://doi.org/10.1007/s00064-019-0605-9.
22. Savvidou OD, Kaspiris A, Goumenos S, Trikoupis I, Melissaridou D, Kalogeropoulos A, Serenidis D, Georgoulis JD, Lianou I, Koulouvaris P, Papagelopoulos PJ. Knee arthrodesis with a modular silver-coated endoprosthesis for infected Total knee arthroplasty with extensive bone loss: a retrospective case-series study. J Clin Med. 2023;12(10):3600. https://doi.org/10.3390/jcm12103600. PMID: 37240706; PMCID: PMC10218786.
23. Wilding CP, Cooper GA, Freeman AK, Parry MC, Jeys L. Can a silver-coated arthrodesis implant provide a viable alternative to above knee amputation in the unsalvageable, infected total knee arthroplasty? J Arthroplast. 2016;31(11):2542–7. https://doi.org/10.1016/j.arth.2016.04.009. Epub 2016 Apr 22
24. Alt V, Heiss C, Rupp M. Treatment of a recurrent Periprosthetic joint infection with an intramedullary knee arthrodesis system with low-amount metallic silver coating. J Bone Jt

Infect. 2019;4(3):111–4. https://doi.org/10.7150/jbji.34484. PMID: 31192109; PMCID: PMC6536804.
25. Balato G, Rizzo M, Ascione T, Smeraglia F, Mariconda M. Re-infection rates and clinical outcomes following arthrodesis with intramedullary nail and external fixator for infected knee prosthesis: a systematic review and meta-analysis. BMC Musculoskelet Disord. 2018;19(1):361. https://doi.org/10.1186/s12891-018-2283-4. PMID: 30301462; PMCID: PMC6178263.
26. Hawi N, Kendoff D, Citak M, Gehrke T, Haasper C. Septic single-stage knee arthrodesis after failed total knee arthroplasty using a cemented coupled nail. Bone Joint J. 2015;97-B(5):649–53. https://doi.org/10.1302/0301-620X.97B5.34902.

Antimicrobial Therapy in One-Stage Revision Surgery

Anna Both, Flaminia Olearo, and Holger Rohde

Introduction and General Concepts

Unlike antibiotic therapy of acute infections caused by rapidly dividing bacteria, anti-infective strategies in PJI have to take into consideration that device-associated infections are associated with specific bacterial phenotypes, i.e., multicellular biofilm formation and intracellular persistence [1, 2]. Generally, biofilm formation is associated with significant changes in bacterial metabolism, ultimately leading to a broadly reduced susceptibility (i.e., increased MICs) against a broad range of antibiotics. Resistance emerging from biofilm formation is unrelated to commonly known specific resistance mechanisms (i.e., expression of defined resistance determinants) and is referred to as phenotypic resistance [3]. Phenotypic resistance, in combination with complex pharmacokinetics present in infected bone and soft tissues and local immune dysfunctions related to the implanted device, demand high doses of systemic as well as topical antibiotics, prolonged therapy courses, and, in some cases, combination therapies.

Duration of Antibiotic Therapy

To date, there is insufficient scientific evidence from randomised clinical trials to make valid recommendations on the optimal duration of treatment for single-stage revision arthroplasty. The majority of available studies on this topic have been conducted in the context of DAIR, and this applies in particular to the few available randomized clinical trials [4, 5]. It is, though, general consent that prolonged antibiotic therapy must be

---

A. Both · F. Olearo · H. Rohde (✉)
Institute for Medical Microbiology, Virology and Hygiene, University Medical Center Hamburg-Eppendorf, Hamburg, Germany
e-mail: a.both@uke.de; f.olearo@uke.de; rohde@uke.de

achieved by combining an initial i.v. therapy course with subsequent oral treatment [6–8]. Thereby, complications (e.g., associated with intravenous catheters) are avoided, and early discharge to rehabilitation facilities is possible. Duration of i.v. treatment is usually 2 weeks, but longer i.v. treatment may be necessary (e.g., PJI caused by *Enterococcus spp.*). Recent evidence indicates that early switch to oral antibiotics is noninferior to six weeks intravenous antibiotic therapy [9], suggesting that two weeks of intravenous antibiotics after surgery may not be necessary in all cases.

Recommendations for oral sequential therapy duration are, however, inconclusive, and greatly differ. While some advocate oral antibiotics for up to 10 weeks [6, 8, 10], also shorter courses are propagated, depending on the clinical context (duration of infection, soft tissue situation, completeness of infected tissue removal) and type of pathogen [8]. Possibly, shortening of total antibiotic treatment duration may reduce numbers of adverse events and costs [5, 11–13]. However, scientific evidence advocating shorter antibiotics courses, in particular in one-stage revision arthroplasty, is scarce. In a recent systematic review of single-stage revision arthroplasty [14], only two / 21 studies included patients who received antibiotics for a maximum of 2 to 6 weeks. In all other trials, the duration of treatment was at least 12 weeks. A recent meta-analysis stratified by operation modality [15], did not find any difference between shorter and longer antimicrobial therapy (pooled risk ratio 0.71 (95% CI 0.45–1.11)), however, just four studies have been included in this meta-regression and there was no distinction between one—and two-stage revision. The largest randomized clinical trial [5] on antibiotics treatment for PJI did not find a non-inferiority of 6-week versus 12-week of post-surgery antibiotic treatment. Criticisms have highlighted that in a sub-group analysis of just one-stage revision procedures, no difference in the risk of joint reinfection between the two treatment groups would have probably been found [16] if the study would have been powered for this analysis, underpinning the urgent need for randomized clinical trials focusing on groups undergoing defined surgical procedures.

Systemic Antibiotics: Options and Limitations

General Considerations

The mainstay of antibiotic i.v. treatment are cell wall active β-lactam antibiotics. They have proven clinical efficacy in infections caused by Gram-positive and-negative bacteria, and also in the context of PJI. A summary of first line compounds recommended for the most relevant pathogens encountered in prosthetic joint infections is given in Tables 1 and 2. Here, also alternatives in case of β-lactam hypersensitivity or detection of acquired resistance mechanisms (e.g., oxacillin-resistance in *S. aureus*, glycopeptide-resistance in *Enterococcus* sp., third generation cephalosporin resistance in *Enterobacterales*) are included. With the emergence and spread of multidrug resistant Gram-negative organisms [MROs, i.e., carbapenem-resistant *Enterobacterales*, carbapenem-resistant non-fermenters (e.g. *Pseudomonas aeruginosa, Acinetobacter baumannii*)] is appears

Table 1 Antibiotics to treat Gram-positive organisms during one-stage revision arthroplasty

Species	Initial i.v. therapy		Sequential therapy	
	First line	Alternatives (e.g. resistance, in tolerance)	First line	Alternatives
Methicillin-susceptible S. aureus (MSSA) or CoNS	Flucloxacillin + rifampin	Cefazolin + rifampin	Levofloxacin or moxifloxacin + rifampin	Clindamycin + rifampin or Cotrimoxazole + rifampin or Linezolid [a] + rifampin
Methicillin-resistant S. aureus (MRSA) or CoNS	Vancomycin + rifampin	Daptomycin [b] + rifampin or fosfomycin	Levofloxacin or moxifloxacin + rifampin	Clindamycin + rifampin or Cotrimoxazole + rifampin or Linezolid [a] + rifampin
E. faecalis	Ampicillin [c] + Ceftriaxone	Vancomycin + gentamicin	Amoxicillin	Linezolid or Dalbavancin
E. faecium	Vancomycin + Gentamicin	Daptomycin [b] + fosfomycin	Linezolid [a]	Dalbavancin
Viridans streptococci	Benzylpenicillin + Gentamicin [d]	Ceftriaxone	Amoxicillin	Clindamycin or Moxifloxacin
β-Hemolytic streptococci	Benzylpenicillin	Ceftriaxone	Amoxicillin	Clindamycin
Cutibacterium spp.	Benzylpenicillin	Ceftriaxone	Amoxicillin	Clindamycin

[a]Note: mandatory monitoring of linezolid side effect in treatment longer than 28 days
[b]Note: Daptomycin dosage 10–12 mg/kg body weight
[c]Note: High dose necessary (12 g/d)
[d]Note: gentamicin may be added according to principles of endocarditis treatment and depending on penicillin MIC [77]

Table 2 Antibiotics to treat Gram-negative organisms during one-stage revision arthroplasty

Species	Initial i.v. therapy		Sequential therapy (oral)	
	First line	Alternatives (e.g. resistance, allergy, intolerance)	First line	Alternatives
Enterobacterales	Ceftriaxone	Meropenem or Ciprofloxacin	Ciprofloxacin	Cotrimoxazole
P. aeruginosa	Ceftazidim + ciprofloxacin or Aminoglycoside	Meropenem or Ciprofloxacin or Ceftolozane-tazobactam	Ciprofloxacin	None [a]
A. baumannii	Carbapenem	None [a]	Ciprofloxacin	None [a]

[a]Note: if carbapenem—and/or ciprofloxacin is tested resistant involvement of PJI referral center recommended. One-stage revision arthroplasty discouraged

plausible to assume that these organisms will become more relevant in PJI in the future. Although some therapeutic options have become available (e.g., ceftazidime-avibactam, ceftolozane-tazobactam, cefiderocol), at present only limited clinical experience is available. Therefore, PJI caused by MROs are defined as difficult to treat [10] and thus qualify for two—rather than one-stage revision procedures. Similarly, PJI caused by fungi are usually defined as difficult to treat and treated using two-stage approaches [8].

Choosing antibiotics for (usually long-term) oral treatment can be challenging. This relates to pharmacokinetic issues (i.e., oral bioavailability), the prevalence of resistant isolates (e.g., lincosamide-resistance in *Staphylococcus spp.*, quinolone-resistance in *Enterobacterales* and *P. aeruginosa*) as well as side effects (e.g., tendinopathies, QT interval prolongation, or neurologic adverse events associated with fluoroquinolones) and interaction profiles (e.g., linezolid interactions with serotonin reuptake inhibitors, induction of cytochrome P450 by rifampin).

Antibiotics therapy in one-stage revision arthroplasty must be initiated only after suitable specimens for microbiological analysis and pathogen detection have been collected. In acute infections (i.e., infections caused by highly virulent pathogens), immediate start of i.v. treatment may then be necessary prior to pathogen identification. Suitable compounds should cover, e.g., *S. aureus*, β-hemolytic streptococci, and *Enterobacterales*, and thus must have Gram-positive and -negative coverage. In selected cases, cerfuroxim (1500 mg q.i.d.) or aminopenicillins-β-lactamase inhibitor combinations (e.g., ampicillin-sulbactam 4000 mg t.i.d.) are possible alternatives. As, however, usually β-lactam resistant organism should also be covered (i.e., methicillin-resistant staphylococci) a practical approach is to combine vancomycin and a Gram-negative active compound (e.g., ceftriaxone). Care should then be taken to optimize treatment as soon as results from microbiological analysis become available.

Importance of Novel Antibiotics in One-Stage Exchange Arthroplasty

As outlined above, several commonly employed i.v. and oral antibiotics are associated with significant issues, e.g., related to drug safety and antimicrobial activity. The approval of new antibiotics over the past years has at least partially increased the number of available drugs with potential importance for PJI treatment, e.g., those caused by staphylococci or enterococci. Importantly, the use of these antibiotics in PJI treatment is usually off-label. Nevertheless, certain characteristics that will be discussed below make them interesting or even necessary alternatives to current standard compounds.

Daptomycin

Daptomycin is a lipopeptide antibiotic approved for the treatment of complicated skin and soft tissue infections, right heart endocarditis, and associated bacteremia caused by *S. aureus* [17]. In a process that has not been fully elucidated, daptomycin interacts with phospholipids of the cell membrane of Gram-positive pathogens and leads to growth-independent cell death by depolarization [18, 19]. Interaction with specific phospholipids explains its exclusive action against Gram-positive pathogens, including the difficult-to-treat methicillin-resistant staphylococci (MRSA) and vancomycin-resistant enterococci (VRE). Importantly, while daptomycin was approved for 4–6 mg/kg body weight in adults, numerous subsequent clinical and experimental studies demonstrated improved efficacy and prevention of resistance development in bloodstream infections and endocarditis caused by MRSA and VRE when used at higher doses of 9–12 mg/kg body weight [20, 21].

To date, no randomized clinical trials to test clinical efficiency daptomycin in the treatment of JI are available, but experimental studies and case series of its use in orthopedic infections appear promising. A retrospective analysis of patients with foreign-material-associated orthopedic infections showed cure rates of 81% in PJI and 86% in other foreign-material-associated osteomyelitis [22]. A meta-analysis which included doses between 4 and 12 mg/kg body weight found cure rates of 70 and 78% in foreign material and non-foreign material associated bone and joint infections, respectively [23].

In PJI, daptomycin is usually used as an alternative to vancomycin in patients with impaired renal function, or side effects related to glycopeptide use. Though data is still relatively scarce, in blood stream infections daptomycin does not appear inferior to vancomycin in terms of mortality [24]. Importantly, adverse events warranting antibiotic discontinuation were rarer in patients receiving daptomycin. However, care must be taken to monitor for serious adverse events like myopathy, rhabdomyolysis, and eosinophilic pneumonia. Indeed, myopathy may occur in up to 14% of patients receiving daptomycin. While patients with reduced kidney function, statin use and obesity are at an increased risk for adverse events, all patients should be monitored for clinical signs of myopathy and creatine phosphokinase elevation [25].

Interestingly, in experimental and early clinical studies combination regimens with fosfomycin [26], ceftaroline [27] or rifampin [28] seem to be more effective than daptomycin alone.

In conclusion, daptomycin is a promising antibiotic for treatment of Gram-positive PJI, especially in patients who cannot tolerate vancomycin. More studies are needed to establish an optimal regimen for PJI, which will most likely include a second antibiotic like rifampin or fosfomycin for combination therapy.

Tigecycline

Tigecycline is a glycylcycline antibiotic derived from minocycline. Tigecycline acts through binding to the 30S ribosomal subunit, inhibiting entry of tRNAs and subsequently protein biosynthesis. It was specifically developed to overcome the major tetracycline resistance mechanisms, namely efflux and ribosomal protection. It has broad activity against both aerobic and anaerobic Gram-positive and Gram-negative bacteria, with the notable exception of *P. aeruginosa*. It is approved by the

FDA and EMA for the treatment of complicated skin and skin structure infections, community-acquired pneumonia and complicated intra-abdominal infections [29, 30].

The primary use of tigecycline is the treatment of polymicrobial infections especially with involvement of extensively drug resistant Gram-negative bacteria [31]. Tigecycline has a large volume of distribution. This pharmacokinetic property makes it an interesting substance for the treatment of bone infections. Though studies on its effectiveness in PJI are largely lacking and limited to case series with very heterogeneous patient cases, in vivo pharmacokinetic studies show promising enrichment in bone. Indeed one study with healthy volunteers showed a bone-to-serum AUC ratio of 4.77 after three doses of tigecycline, using the recommended dosing interval, providing evidence for bone penetration [32].

Interestingly, in a clinical trial comparing once daily tigecycline to ertapenem +/− vancomycin for diabetic foot infection, tigecycline did not meet non-inferiority criteria. It is not entirely clear why this was the case. Possibly a lack of pre-treatment assessment of osteomyelitis may have led to too-short courses of tigeycline, side effects (mostly nausea and vomiting) prompting a switch from tigecycline to a different drug may have played a role and in the study a higher breakpoint for susceptibility (≤ 2 mg/L) were accepted [33]. However, overall lower effectiveness of tigecycline in deep tissue infections including osteomyelitis is possible and tigecycline is currently not first choice in osteomyelitis or PJI. However, tigecycline can be an important asset in the context of infections caused by extensively drug resistant (XDR) pathogens. It has been used for treatment of XDR *Klebsiella pneumoniae*, *Escherichia coli*, and *Acinetobacter baumannii*, but MIC interpretation is difficult in many species and the determination of an optimal treatment plan requires expertise. A microbiologist or infectious disease specialist should be consulted in these cases, since high dose regimens and combination therapy may be more likely to result in clinical cure [34–36].

Linezolid

Linezolid is an oxazolidinone antibiotic, which is bacteriostatic by inhibiting the initiation of protein synthesis at the 50S ribosomal subunit. It has broad spectrum activity against Gram-positive bacteria, including Methicillin-resistant staphylococci and vancomycin-resistant enterococci. It is FDA and EMA approved for treatment of pneumonia and skin and skin structure infections [30].

Due to its excellent bioavailability and activity against multi-drug resistant Gram-positive bacteria linezolid has received some interest for the treatment of PJI. However, its long-term use is limited by potentially severe adverse effects, such as myelosuppression, lactic acidosis, and optical and peripheral neurotoxicity and generally use for more than 28 days is not recommended.

Thrombocytopenia is the most common presentation of linezolid-induced myelosuppression and may occur in around 30% of patients who receive linezolid for >10d [37]. Neuropathy is also strikingly dependent on treatment duration. The use of linezolid in the treatment of extensively resistant tuberculosis has garnered some experience with prolonged use, showing up to 58% of patients suffering from peripheral or optical neuropathy after a mean treatment duration of 13 months [38].

Besides duration of therapy, renal impairment is a risk factors for adverse events [39]. Even though no dose adjustment according to renal function is recommended at present, therapeutic drug monitoring may be warranted in special patient populations, such as patients with renal impairment, adipositas or under ICU care.

While patients usually recover from myelosuppression 1–3 weeks after discontinuation of linezolid therapy, neuropathy may be permanent and linezolid-induced lactic acidosis—though rare—has a mortality of 25% [40–42].

So far there are no randomized controlled trials of the efficacy and safety of linezolid in PJI. However, observational studies have assessed its use in this indication. A 2020 systematic review including 372 patients with PJI treated with linezolid alone or in combination report control of infection in 80% of cases (range 30–100%), but definitions of infection, indication for linezolid therapy, combinations with other antibiotic agents and surgical approach were heterogeneous [43].

In clinical practice, combination therapy with rifampin is commonly used [43]. However, there is no data showing the superiority of the combination over linezolid alone and there is concern over increased toxicity and drug interactions, which may lead to insufficient linezolid concentrations [44].

Overall, prospective clinical studies with homogeneous case definitions are urgently needed to clearly assess the usefulness of linezolid in the treatment of PJI. For now, the available data quality is insufficient and thus, linezolid is recommended only as second line drug in difficult-to-treat gram-positive organisms and stress the importance of patient consent and close monitoring in applying linezolid for PJI antibiotic therapy.

In conclusion, linezolid may be a suitable agent in PJI cases with difficult to treat organisms, such as enterococci. It is not licensed for use beyond 28 days and the advantages of linezolid therapy, such as early switch to oral therapy in difficult-to-treat pathogens, against the risk of possibly important and irreversible side effects. In any case, the use of linezolid beyond 28 days warrants monitoring of treatment-associated adverse effects.

Dalbavancin

Dalbavancin is a bactericidal lipoglycopeptide antibiotic, related to vancomycin. It inhibits bacterial cell wall biosynthesis by binding to the terminal D-alanyl-D-alanine of the peptidoglycan precursor. Because of this mechanism of action, it is only active against Gram-positive pathogens, like *S. aureus* and *Streptococcus* sp. (including difficult-to-treat organisms, e.g., MRSA). In vitro studies have even shown activity against vancomycin-resistant enterococci (VRE), which carried a *vanB* resistance determinant. However, the activity against VRE remains to be properly assessed in clinical studies. Importantly, *vanA*-positive VRE showed resistance against dalbavancin.

Lipoglycopeptides show a prolonged half-life, and the estimated terminal dalbavancin half-life is approximately 14.5 days. This allows for a convenient dosing regimen, which may facilitate patient adherence and allow for outpatient management [45, 46]. Currently, dalbavancin is approved by the FDA and EMA for treatment of acute skin and soft tissue infections (SSTI) caused by susceptible organisms. For this indication, the recommended dose is a single infusion of 1500 mg or two divides doses of 1000 mg and 500 mg 1 week apart. For the indication of acute SSTI, dalbavancin showed non-inferiority against vancomycin and linezolid. Of note, adverse events were shown to be significantly less common in dalbavancin compared to vancomycin, linezolid, and daptomycin [47]. The convenient dosing and favorable risk profile, combined with its broad spectrum of activity makes dalbavancin an interesting substance for use in prosthetic joint infections, especially for outpatient care settings. Unfortunately, prospective trials assessing its efficacy in PJI have not yet been conducted. A recent review of the literature from 2021 finds a cure rate of 73% over all published PJI cases treated with dalbavancin [48]. However, published cure rates varied widely between 33 and 90%, and treatment regimens were very heterogeneous, including dosing. Indeed, dosing of dalbavancin in PJI is not yet standardized. A phase I study assessed dalbavancin levels in bone, synovium, and plasma at different time points and across different doses. It found concentrations relevant for the treatment of osteomyelitis in bone and surrounding tissues. Pharmacokinetic modeling suggested a similar AUC over MIC in both a regimen of 1500 mg i.v. given twice, 1 week apart and a 1000 mg initial dose, followed by 4 weekly doses of 500 mg [49]. Data from animal studies suggest that regimens with larger initial doses with wider dosing intervals were more efficacious in bone infection compared to smaller but closer spaced ones [50]. Pending further studies in relevant clinical cohorts, based on the data available, employing a dosing of 1500 mg on day 1 and day 8 in PJI patients appears appropriate. Dalbavancin treatment is usually started after 1–2 weeks of inpatient treatment with conventional intravenous antibiotic regimens. When selecting patients who may benefit from dalbavancin, the following factors are of primary importance: staphylococci or streptococci with resistance against other orally available antibiotics (e.g., fluorquinolones, clindamycin), adverse effects from other antibiotics with Gram-positive coverage, and broad spectrum activity in mixed infection with Gram-positive bacteria. In conclusion, dalbavancin is a promising new agent in the treatment of PJI.

The Role of Combination Therapies in One-Stage Revision Arthroplasty

Several rationales encourage combination of two or more antibiotics in clinical practice, e.g., achievement of broad pathogen coverage in empirical treatment settings, sufficient coverage in polymicrobial infections, and reduction of antibiotic resistance development [51]. The interaction between two antibiotics can have synergistic, antagonistic, additive, or indifferent effects. Clinically relevant examples for synergisms are combination of ceftriaxone and ampicillin to treat *E. faecalis* [52, 53], or antipseudomonal cephalosporins and aminoglycosides (e.g., amikacin) to treat *P. aeruginosa* infections [54]. In PJI, related to the presence of slow growing, antibiotic tolerant bacterial populations, achievement of antibiotic synergism has been explored to overcome phenotypic resistance. It needs to be stressed, though, that current evidence from clinical studies does not advocate combination therapy in all types of PJI, but directs in particular toward its use in staphylococcal infections.

Rifampin is considered the cornerstone of the antimicrobial treatment for PJI caused by *S. aureus* or Coagulase-negative staphylococci. It has excellent activity against staphylococci and exerts a particularly noteworthy activity against slow growing bacteria embedded in a biofilm consortium. However, during monotherapy, resistance is rapidly developing by a single point mutation within the DNA-dependent RNA polymerase-encoding *rpoB* gene. For this reason, rifampin strictly may only be used in combination therapies, e.g., combined with β-lactam antibiotics [55], quinolones [4, 56], fusidic acid [57], linezolid [58], vancomycin [59], or clindamycin [60]. In fact, an early, randomized controlled trial (RCT) [56] showed that the combination of fluorquinolones with rifampin achieved a clinical success of DAIR procedure for PJI treatment of 100% (12/12 patients) compared to ciprofloxacin monotherapy, which was associated with a failure rate of 42%. Another RCT found that high clinical success rate was maintained even with a shorter treatment (8-weeks levofloxacin-rifampin combination) compared to 3–6 months of the same regimen [4] (difference 3.3%, 95% CI −11.7–18.3%). Recently, the combination moxifloxacin and rifampin has been preferred over the other quinolone for MSSA PJI because of the higher genetic barrier for resistance development [61].

Although promising in vitro studies encouraged the combination linezolid with rifampin [62], the absence of controlled head-to-head studies comparing linezolid monotherapy and its combination with rifampin [63] and serum linezolid levels drop under rifampin therapy [64, 65], suggest to employ this combination with precautions and to monitor linezolid serum levels.

Rifampin is a potent inducer of both cytochrome P-450 oxidative enzymes and the P-glycoprotein transport system [66], thereby causing potential life-threatening drug–drug interactions, especially in the elderly population and immunosuppressed patients. For this reason, the key role of rifampin for staphylococcal PJI [67] has been challenged in two recent systematic reviews with meta-analysis [68, 69]. While the study of Aydin et al. [68] found no evidence to encourage rifampin combination therapy for staphylococcal PJI, Scheper et al. [69] found just a marginal improvement of 10% success rate for staphylococcal prosthetic knee infections. Available studies were, although, hampered by confounding, selection, and publication bias, precluding conclusive statements on the role of rifampin in PJI treatment. RCTs are urgently needed to evaluate the exact clinical benefit of rifampin combination therapy in staphylococcal PJI. Possibly, rifampin-free combinations may replace current strategies in staphylococcal PJI treatment. For example, ceftobiprol or fosfomycin with daptomycin have been shown to exhibit synergistic effects in vitro and pre-clinical in vivo models of PJI [70–72].

Compared to staphylococcal PJI, evidence for the use of combination therapy in PJI caused by other Gram-positive pathogens is scarce. Importantly, transfer of recommendations available for other biofilm-associated infections, e.g., infective endocarditis (IE), is difficult. For example, the combination of vancomycin or beta-lactams with aminoglycosides for treatment of *E. faecalis* IE did not show any advantage compared to the monotherapy for enterococcal PJIs [73]. On the other hand the synergism between ceftriaxone and ampicillin, standard of care for *E. faecalis* endocarditis, has shown encouraging outcomes for *E. faecalis* PJIs [74], although clinical data are scarce [75]. Nevertheless, the combination of ampicillin and ceftriaxone has been adopted as standard treatment for *E. faecalis* PJI in many centers.

Viridans streptococci are another important group of Gram-positive, PJI-causing pathogens for which combination of benzylpenicillin and gentamicin recommended for PJI treatment. This combination is also used in IE treatment, based on the synergistic antibiotic activity against planktonic and biofilm-forming *Streptococcus* spp. in vitro [76]. The addition of gentamicin is usually reserved for infections caused by *Streptococcus* sp. Isolates with penicillin MICs $\geq 0.25–2$ mg/L [77]. Intriguing, rifampin may substitute gentamicin as a combination partner [78], however, at present available evidence does not advocate this is not strong enough [68].

Also for *Enterobacterales* and non-fermenters, available evidence to support the use of combination therapies in PJI is scarce. Some pre-clinical studies suggest that possibly, combinations (e.g., fluorquinolons with fosfomycin) may be superior compared to mono therapy [79–81]. At present, however, this assumption are based on few clinical studies with no focus on just PJI and not stratified by infection causing pathogens. In the future, the emergence of infections caused by multidrug resistant isolates (e.g., carbapenemase-producing *Enterobacterales*, carbapenem-resistant *P. aeruginosa* or *A. baumannii*) may change the current role of combination therapies.

Local Antibiotics

Related to reduced perfusion caused by infection itself and as a consequence of surgical procedures, accessibility of i.v. antibiotics to the infection site may be limited. In single stage surgery, this apparently increases the risk of implant colonization by bacteria that were not removed during surgical debridement. A strategy to overcome this problem is to install local antibiotics. The achievement of exceedingly high local antibiotics levels is thought to suppress bacterial growth or even kill residual pathogens during the time window needed to establish sufficiently high tissue levels by i.v. antibiotic treatment. Usually this is achieved by the release of antibiotics, added to bone cement preparations (referred to as antibiotic loaded cement, ALC).

In fact, evidence shows that the use of ALC is able to reduce infection rates during primary arthroplasty, supporting the idea that local antibiotics may serve as a mean to protect implanted material from bacterial colonization [82]. Therefore, combination of systemic i.v. with ALC is a standard approach in one-stage revision arthroplasty.

Table 3 Antibiotics useful for custom preparations of antibiotics loaded bone cement

Drug	Concentration (per 40 g cement)	Application (examples for specific pathogens)
Daptomycin	1 g	Vancomycin-resistant *Enterococcus* sp.
Meropenem	2 g	Enterobacterales/*P. aeruginosa*
Colistin[a]	12 Mio—24 Mio IU (equals 1–2 g CMS[a])	Carbapenem-resistant organisms
Amphotericin B[b]	200 mg	Yeast

[a] 12.500 IU/mg Colistinmethatsodium (CMS); 1 Mio IU = 80 mg CMS = 32 mg Colisitin base (CBA)
[b] Liposomal preparations (e.g., Ambisome, Gilead)

To this end, antibiotics (products approved for i.v. use) can be added to available commercial bone cement preparations (e.g., Palacos, Simplex). It needs to be underpinned, however, that custom preparation of ALC may cause problems, e.g., reduced stability and insufficient antibiotics release can result from inhomogeneous mixing. In addition, modification of commercial products by addition of antibiotics causes issues related to medico legal regulations. Therefore, if ever possible, the use of commercially available, fixed cement-antibiotics preparations (e.g., Copal G + C [contains gentamicin and clindamycin; Haereus, Wehrheim, Germany], Simplex + tobramycin [Stryker, Duisburg, Germany) is strongly encouraged.

In some cases, however, commercial solutions do not cover PJI-causing organisms in individual patient (e.g., resistance against in-built antibiotics, infections caused by multi-resistant bacteria or fungi). Under these circumstances, manual addition of antibiotics is necessary. Here, strict recognition of sufficient compound stability (e.g., against higher temperatures occurring during polymerization) as well as experimental evidence for its release from bone cement is mandatory [82]. Moreover, the total concentration of added antibiotics must not exceed 10% (wt/wt) to not cause mechanical instability of the product [82]. Table 3 provides an overview over antibiotics and antifungals which are currently under use as additives to bone cement preparations, possible concentrations and indications.

References

1. Beam E, Osmon D. Prosthetic joint infection update. Infect Dis Clin N Am. 2018;32(4):843–59.
2. Saeed K, McLaren AC, Schwarz EM, Antoci V, Arnold WV, Chen AF, et al. 2018 international consensus meeting on musculoskeletal infection: summary from the biofilm workgroup and consensus on biofilm related musculoskeletal infections. J Orthop Res. 2019;37(5):1007–17.
3. Lamret F, Colin M, Mongaret C, Gangloff SC, Reffuveille F. Antibiotic tolerance of Staphylococcus aureus biofilm in periprosthetic joint infections and Antibiofilm strategies. Antibiotics (Basel). 2020;9(9):547.
4. Lora-Tamayo J, Euba G, Cobo J, Horcajada JP, Soriano A, Sandoval E, et al. Short—versus long-duration levofloxacin plus rifampicin for acute staphylococcal prosthetic joint infection managed with implant retention: a randomised clinical trial. Int J Antimicrob Agents. 2016;48(3):310–6.

5. Bernard L, Arvieux C, Brunschweiler B, Touchais S, Ansart S, Bru JP, et al. Antibiotic therapy for 6 or 12 weeks for prosthetic joint infection. N Engl J Med. 2021;384(21):1991–2001.
6. Osmon DR, Berbari EF, Berendt AR, Lew D, Zimmerli W, Steckelberg JM, et al. Executive summary: diagnosis and management of prosthetic joint infection: clinical practice guidelines by the Infectious Diseases Society of America. Clin Infect Dis. 2013;56(1):1–10.
7. Parvizi J, Adeli B, Zmistowski B, Restrepo C, Greenwald AS. Management of periprosthetic joint infection: the current knowledge: AAOS exhibit selection. J Bone Joint Surg Am. 2012;94(14):e104.
8. Ometti M, Delmastro E, Salini V. Management of prosthetic joint infections: a guidelines comparison. Musculoskelet Surg. 2022;106(3):219–26.
9. Li HK, Rombach I, Zambellas R, Walker AS, McNally MA, Atkins BL, et al. Oral versus intravenous antibiotics for bone and joint infection. N Engl J Med. 2019;380(5):425–36.
10. Zijlstra WP, Ploegmakers JJW, Kampinga GA, Toren-Wielema ML, Ettema HB, Knobben BAS, et al. A protocol for periprosthetic joint infections from the northern infection network for joint arthroplasty (NINJA) in The Netherlands. Arthroplasty. 2022;4(1):19.
11. Lesens O, Ferry T, Forestier E, Botelho-Nevers E, Pavese P, Piet E, et al. Should we expand the indications for the DAIR (debridement, antibiotic therapy, and implant retention) procedure for Staphylococcus aureus prosthetic joint infections? A multicenter retrospective study. Eur J Clin Microbiol Infect Dis. 2018;37(10):1949–56.
12. Esposito S, Esposito I, Leone S. Considerations of antibiotic therapy duration in community—and hospital-acquired bacterial infections. J Antimicrob Chemother. 2012;67(11):2570–5.
13. Duggal A, Barsoum W, Schmitt SK. Patients with prosthetic joint infection on IV antibiotics are at high risk for readmission. Clin Orthop Relat Res. 2009;467(7):1727–31.
14. Sandiford NA, McHale A, Citak M, Kendoff D. What is the optimal duration of intravenous antibiotics following single-stage revision total hip arthroplasty for prosthetic joint infection? A systematic review. Hip Int. 2021;31(3):286–94.
15. Yen HT, Hsieh RW, Huang CY, Hsu TC, Yeh T, Chen YC, et al. Short-course versus long-course antibiotics in prosthetic joint infections: a systematic review and meta-analysis of one randomized controlled trial plus nine observational studies. J Antimicrob Chemother. 2019;74(9):2507–16.
16. Di Matteo B, Marcacci M. Antibiotic therapy for 6 or 12 weeks for prosthetic joint infection. N Engl J Med. 2022;386(10):1001–2.
17. Johnson A. Daptomycin in the treatment of skin, soft-tissue and invasive infections due to gram-positive bacteria. Future Microbiol. 2006;1(3):255–65.
18. Miller WR, Bayer AS, Arias CA. Mechanism of action and resistance to Daptomycin in Staphylococcus aureus and enterococci. Cold Spring Harb Perspect Med. 2016;6(11):a026997.
19. Humphries RM, Pollett S, Sakoulas G. A current perspective on daptomycin for the clinical microbiologist. Clin Microbiol Rev. 2013;26(4):759–80.
20. Foolad F, Taylor BD, Shelburne SA, Arias CA, Aitken SL. Association of daptomycin dosing regimen and mortality in patients with VRE bacteraemia: a review. J Antimicrob Chemother. 2018;73(9):2277–83.
21. Smith JR, Claeys KC, Barber KE, Rybak MJ. High-dose daptomycin therapy for staphylococcal endocarditis and when to apply it. Curr Infect Dis Rep. 2014;16(10):429.
22. Hermsen ED, Mendez-Vigo L, Berbari EF, Chung T, Yoon M, Lamp KC. A retrospective study of outcomes of device-associated osteomyelitis treated with daptomycin. BMC Infect Dis. 2016;16:310.
23. Telles JP, Cieslinski J, Tuon FF. Daptomycin to bone and joint infections and prosthesis joint infections: a systematic review. Braz J Infect Dis. 2019;23(3):191–6.
24. Maraolo AE, Giaccone A, Gentile I, Saracino A, Bavaro DF. Daptomycin versus vancomycin for the treatment of methicillin-resistant Staphylococcus aureus bloodstream infection with or without endocarditis: a systematic review and meta-analysis. Antibiotics (Basel). 2021;10(8):1014.
25. Dare RK, Tewell C, Harris B, Wright PW, Van Driest SL, Farber-Eger E, et al. Effect of statin Coadministration on the risk of Daptomycin-associated myopathy. Clin Infect Dis. 2018;67(9):1356–63.

26. Pujol M, Miro JM, Shaw E, Aguado JM, San-Juan R, Puig-Asensio M, et al. Daptomycin plus Fosfomycin versus Daptomycin alone for methicillin-resistant Staphylococcus aureus bacteremia and endocarditis: a randomized clinical trial. Clin Infect Dis. 2021;72(9):1517–25.
27. Geriak M, Haddad F, Rizvi K, Rose W, Kullar R, LaPlante K, et al. Clinical data on Daptomycin plus Ceftaroline versus standard of care monotherapy in the treatment of methicillin-resistant Staphylococcus aureus bacteremia. Antimicrob Agents Chemother. 2019;63(5):e02483–18.
28. Lefebvre M, Jacqueline C, Amador G, Le Mabecque V, Miegeville A, Potel G, et al. Efficacy of daptomycin combined with rifampicin for the treatment of experimental meticillin-resistant Staphylococcus aureus (MRSA) acute osteomyelitis. Int J Antimicrob Agents. 2010;36(6):542–4.
29. Falagas ME, Metaxas EI. Tigecycline for the treatment of patients with community-acquired pneumonia requiring hospitalization. Expert Rev Anti-Infect Ther. 2009;7(8):913–23.
30. Barton E, MacGowan A. Future treatment options for Gram-positive infections—looking ahead. Clin Microbiol Infect. 2009;15(Suppl 6):17–25.
31. Yaghoubi S, Zekiy AO, Krutova M, Gholami M, Kouhsari E, Sholeh M, et al. Tigecycline antibacterial activity, clinical effectiveness, and mechanisms and epidemiology of resistance: narrative review. Eur J Clin Microbiol Infect Dis. 2022;41(7):1003–22.
32. Bhattacharya I, Gotfried MH, Ji AJ, Saunders JP, Gourley I, Diehl A, et al. Reassessment of tigecycline bone concentrations in volunteers undergoing elective orthopedic procedures. J Clin Pharmacol. 2014;54(1):70–4.
33. Lauf L, Ozsvar Z, Mitha I, Regoly-Merei J, Embil JM, Cooper A, et al. Phase 3 study comparing tigecycline and ertapenem in patients with diabetic foot infections with and without osteomyelitis. Diagn Microbiol Infect Dis. 2014;78(4):469–80.
34. Gong J, Su D, Shang J, Yu H, Du G, Lin Y, et al. Efficacy and safety of high-dose tigecycline for the treatment of infectious diseases: a meta-analysis. Medicine (Baltimore). 2019;98(38):e17091.
35. Cai Y, Bai N, Liu X, Liang B, Wang J, Wang R. Tigecycline: alone or in combination? Infect Dis (Lond). 2016;48(7):491–502.
36. EUCAST. https://www.eucast.org/fileadmin/src/media/PDFs/EUCAST_files/Guidance_documents/Tigecycline_Guidance_document_v2_20220720.pdf.
37. Attassi K, Hershberger E, Alam R, Zervos MJ. Thrombocytopenia associated with linezolid therapy. Clin Infect Dis. 2002;34(5):695–8.
38. Jaspard M, Butel N, El Helali N, Marigot-Outtandy D, Guillot H, Peytavin G, et al. Linezolid-associated neurologic adverse events in patients with multidrug-resistant tuberculosis, France. Emerg Infect Dis. 2020;26(8):1792–800.
39. Dai Y, Jiang S, Chen X, Han L, Zhang C, Yu X, et al. Analysis of the risk factors of linezolid-related haematological toxicity in Chinese patients. J Clin Pharm Ther. 2021;46(3):807–13.
40. Gerson SL, Kaplan SL, Bruss JB, Le V, Arellano FM, Hafkin B, et al. Hematologic effects of linezolid: summary of clinical experience. Antimicrob Agents Chemother. 2002;46(8):2723–6.
41. Green SL, Maddox JC, Huttenbach ED. Linezolid and reversible myelosuppression. JAMA. 2001;285(10):1291.
42. Mao Y, Dai D, Jin H, Wang Y. The risk factors of linezolid-induced lactic acidosis: a case report and review. Medicine (Baltimore). 2018;97(36):e12114.
43. Theil C, Schmidt-Braekling T, Gosheger G, Schwarze J, Dieckmann R, Schneider KN, et al. Clinical use of linezolid in periprosthetic joint infections—a systematic review. J Bone Jt Infect. 2020;6(1):7–16.
44. Gandelman K, Zhu T, Fahmi OA, Glue P, Lian K, Obach RS, et al. Unexpected effect of rifampin on the pharmacokinetics of linezolid: in silico and in vitro approaches to explain its mechanism. J Clin Pharmacol. 2011;51(2):229–36.
45. Smith JR, Roberts KD, Rybak MJ. Dalbavancin: a novel Lipoglycopeptide antibiotic with extended activity against gram-positive infections. Infect Dis Ther. 2015;4(3):245–58.
46. Leighton A, Gottlieb AB, Dorr MB, Jabes D, Mosconi G, VanSaders C, et al. Tolerability, pharmacokinetics, and serum bactericidal activity of intravenous dalbavancin in healthy volunteers. Antimicrob Agents Chemother. 2004;48(3):940–5.

47. Guest JF, Esteban J, Manganelli AG, Novelli A, Rizzardini G, Serra M. Comparative efficacy and safety of antibiotics used to treat acute bacterial skin and skin structure infections: results of a network meta-analysis. PLoS One. 2017;12(11):e0187792.
48. Matt M, Duran C, Courjon J, Lotte R, Moing VL, Monnin B, et al. Dalbavancin treatment for prosthetic joint infections in real-life: a national cohort study and literature review. J Glob Antimicrob Resist. 2021;25:341–5.
49. Dunne MW, Puttagunta S, Sprenger CR, Rubino C, Van Wart S, Baldassarre J. Extended-duration dosing and distribution of dalbavancin into bone and articular tissue. Antimicrob Agents Chemother. 2015;59(4):1849–55.
50. Andes D, Craig WA. In vivo pharmacodynamic activity of the glycopeptide dalbavancin. Antimicrob Agents Chemother. 2007;51(5):1633–42.
51. Samuel JR, Gould FK. Prosthetic joint infections: single versus combination therapy. J Antimicrob Chemother. 2010;65(1):18–23.
52. Marino A, Munafo A, Zagami A, Ceccarelli M, Di Mauro R, Cantarella G, et al. Ampicillin plus ceftriaxone regimen against enterococcus faecalis endocarditis: a literature review. J Clin Med. 2021;10(19):4594.
53. Beganovic M, Luther MK, Rice LB, Arias CA, Rybak MJ, LaPlante KL. A review of combination antimicrobial therapy for Enterococcus faecalis bloodstream infections and infective endocarditis. Clin Infect Dis. 2018;67(2):303–9.
54. Baltch AL, Smith RP. Combinations of antibiotics against Pseudomonas aeruginosa. Am J Med. 1985;79(1A):8–16.
55. Zimmerli W, Frei R, Widmer AF, Rajacic Z. Microbiological tests to predict treatment outcome in experimental device-related infections due to Staphylococcus aureus. J Antimicrob Chemother. 1994;33(5):959–67.
56. Zimmerli W, Widmer AF, Blatter M, Frei R, Ochsner PE. Role of rifampin for treatment of orthopedic implant-related staphylococcal infections: a randomized controlled trial. Foreign-body infection (FBI) study group. JAMA. 1998;279(19):1537–41.
57. Drancourt M, Stein A, Argenson JN, Roiron R, Groulier P, Raoult D. Oral treatment of staphylococcus spp. infected orthopaedic implants with fusidic acid or ofloxacin in combination with rifampicin. J Antimicrob Chemother. 1997;39(2):235–40.
58. Jacqueline C, Caillon J, Le Mabecque V, Miegeville AF, Donnio PY, Bugnon D, et al. In vitro activity of linezolid alone and in combination with gentamicin, vancomycin or rifampicin against methicillin-resistant Staphylococcus aureus by time-kill curve methods. J Antimicrob Chemother. 2003;51(4):857–64.
59. Niska JA, Shahbazian JH, Ramos RI, Francis KP, Bernthal NM, Miller LS. Vancomycin-rifampin combination therapy has enhanced efficacy against an experimental Staphylococcus aureus prosthetic joint infection. Antimicrob Agents Chemother. 2013;57(10):5080–6.
60. Leijtens B, Elbers JBW, Sturm PD, Kullberg BJ, Schreurs BW. Clindamycin-rifampin combination therapy for staphylococcal periprosthetic joint infections: a retrospective observational study. BMC Infect Dis. 2017;17(1):321.
61. Wouthuyzen-Bakker M, Tornero E, Morata L, Nannan Panday PV, Jutte PC, Bori G, et al. Moxifloxacin plus rifampin as an alternative for levofloxacin plus rifampin in the treatment of a prosthetic joint infection with Staphylococcus aureus. Int J Antimicrob Agents. 2018;51(1):38–42.
62. Thompson JM, Saini V, Ashbaugh AG, Miller RJ, Ordonez AA, Ortines RV, et al. Oral-only linezolid-rifampin is highly effective compared with other antibiotics for Periprosthetic joint infection: study of a mouse model. J Bone Joint Surg Am. 2017;99(8):656–65.
63. Morata L, Senneville E, Bernard L, Nguyen S, Buzele R, Druon J, et al. A retrospective review of the clinical experience of linezolid with or without rifampicin in prosthetic joint infections treated with debridement and implant retention. Infect Dis Ther. 2014;3(2):235–43.
64. Gebhart BC, Barker BC, Markewitz BA. Decreased serum linezolid levels in a critically ill patient receiving concomitant linezolid and rifampin. Pharmacotherapy. 2007;27(3):476–9.
65. Tornero E, Morata L, Martinez-Pastor JC, Angulo S, Combalia A, Bori G, et al. Importance of selection and duration of antibiotic regimen in prosthetic joint infections treated with debridement and implant retention. J Antimicrob Chemother. 2016;71(5):1395–401.

66. Baciewicz AM, Chrisman CR, Finch CK, Self TH. Update on rifampin, rifabutin, and rifapentine drug interactions. Curr Med Res Opin. 2013;29(1):1–12.
67. Barberan J. Management of infections of osteoarticular prosthesis. Clin Microbiol Infect. 2006;12(Suppl 3):93–101.
68. Aydin O, Ergen P, Ozturan B, Ozkan K, Arslan F, Vahaboglu H. Rifampin-accompanied antibiotic regimens in the treatment of prosthetic joint infections: a frequentist and Bayesian meta-analysis of current evidence. Eur J Clin Microbiol Infect Dis. 2021;40(4):665–71.
69. Scheper H, Gerritsen LM, Pijls BG, Van Asten SA, Visser LG, De Boer MGJ. Outcome of debridement, antibiotics, and implant retention for staphylococcal hip and knee prosthetic joint infections, focused on rifampicin use: a systematic review and meta-analysis. Open Forum Infect Dis. 2021;8(7):ofab298.
70. Rand KH, Houck HJ. Synergy of daptomycin with oxacillin and other beta-lactams against methicillin-resistant Staphylococcus aureus. Antimicrob Agents Chemother. 2004;48(8):2871–5.
71. Barber KE, Werth BJ, Ireland CE, Stone NE, Nonejuie P, Sakoulas G, et al. Potent synergy of ceftobiprole plus daptomycin against multiple strains of Staphylococcus aureus with various resistance phenotypes. J Antimicrob Chemother. 2014;69(11):3006–10.
72. Antonello RM, Principe L, Maraolo AE, Viaggi V, Pol R, Fabbiani M, et al. Fosfomycin as partner drug for systemic infection management. A systematic review of its synergistic properties from in vitro and in vivo studies. Antibiotics (Basel). 2020;9(8):500.
73. El Helou OC, Berbari EF, Marculescu CE, El Atrouni WI, Razonable RR, Steckelberg JM, et al. Outcome of enterococcal prosthetic joint infection: is combination systemic therapy superior to monotherapy? Clin Infect Dis. 2008;47(7):903–9.
74. Euba G, Lora-Tamayo J, Murillo O, Pedrero S, Cabo J, Verdaguer R, et al. Pilot study of ampicillin-ceftriaxone combination for treatment of orthopedic infections due to enterococcus faecalis. Antimicrob Agents Chemother. 2009;53(10):4305–10.
75. Tornero E, Senneville E, Euba G, Petersdorf S, Rodriguez-Pardo D, Lakatos B, et al. Characteristics of prosthetic joint infections due to enterococcus sp. and predictors of failure: a multi-national study. Clin Microbiol Infect. 2014;20(11):1219–24.
76. Gonzalez Moreno M, Trampuz A, Di Luca M. Synergistic antibiotic activity against planktonic and biofilm-embedded Streptococcus agalactiae, streptococcus pyogenes and Streptococcus oralis. J Antimicrob Chemother. 2017;72(11):3085–92.
77. Baddour LM, Wilson WR, Bayer AS, Fowler VG Jr, Tleyjeh IM, Rybak MJ, et al. Infective endocarditis in adults: diagnosis, antimicrobial therapy, and management of complications: a scientific statement for healthcare professionals from the American Heart Association. Circulation. 2015;132(15):1435–86.
78. Fiaux E, Titecat M, Robineau O, Lora-Tamayo J, El Samad Y, Etienne M, et al. Outcome of patients with streptococcal prosthetic joint infections with special reference to rifampicin combinations. BMC Infect Dis. 2016;16(1):568.
79. Benito N, Franco M, Ribera A, Soriano A, Rodriguez-Pardo D, Sorli L, et al. Time trends in the aetiology of prosthetic joint infections: a multicentre cohort study. Clin Microbiol Infect. 2016;22(8):e1–8.
80. Michalopoulos AS, Livaditis IG, Gougoutas V. The revival of fosfomycin. Int J Infect Dis. 2011;15(11):e732–9.
81. Corvec S, Furustrand Tafin U, Betrisey B, Borens O, Trampuz A. Activities of fosfomycin, tigecycline, colistin, and gentamicin against extended-spectrum-beta-lactamase-producing Escherichia coli in a foreign-body infection model. Antimicrob Agents Chemother. 2013;57(3):1421–7.
82. Martinez-Moreno J, Merino V, Nacher A, Rodrigo JL, Climente M, Merino-Sanjuan M. Antibiotic-loaded bone cement as prophylaxis in total joint replacement. Orthop Surg. 2017;9(4):331–41.

Rehabilitation After One-Stage Septic Exchange

Johannes Reich

The objective of rehabilitation after septic exchange is basically similar to the initial one after a hip or knee replacement. Most important is the improvement of the patient's mobility, the alleviation of pain and the improvement of the patient's well-being in general [1, 2]. The same applies to the rehabilitation after a septic exchange. Further objectives, however, have to be determined on an individual basis.

The main difference between the primary provision of medical care is to be seen in a prolonged hospital stay. The average time spent at hospital depends on the one hand on the clinical process of recovery and on the results of the chemical tests, and on the other hand, on the duration of administering antibiotics.

During the whole process of rehabilitation, it is essential to control the intensity of the training impulses so that, weakened after the operation anyway, the patient's recovery will not be impaired unnecessarily. That means that in the early stage of rehabilitation the intensity of the exercises has to be increased gradually and that the ADLS (Activity daily living skills) have to be acquired, always trying to avoid a negative influence on the still vulnerable wound.

As a rule, physiotherapy starts from day one after the operation with one or two exercises a day. At the beginning, the primary aim is the improvement of the blood circulation, the improved mobility of the joint in question and the patient's confidence to be able to stand up and walk. At this stage, the RICE rule (Rest—Ice—Compression—Elevation) should be applied to guarantee a positive healing effect on the joint. Numerous studies, however, do not recommend cryotherapy [3–8]. At least, no significant differences as to the intensity of the pain of the reduction of the use of painkillers could be shown. Some other studies, however, could show a reduction of the blood loss after total hip arthroplasty [9–11]. Patients, however, describe its application as beneficial. The temperature of the skin, however, should

J. Reich (✉)
ENDO Rehabilitation Center GmbH, Hamburg, Germany
e-mail: johannes.reich@helios-gesundheit.de

© The Author(s), under exclusive license to Springer Nature Switzerland AG 2024
M. Citak et al. (eds.), *One-Stage Septic Revision Arthroplasty*,
https://doi.org/10.1007/978-3-031-59160-0_12

not be lowered too far in order to avoid a negative influence on the regeneration of the cells. So only short phases of the application of ice are recommended.

The surgical technique used by the operating team puts certain limits on the patient's mobilization. That applies to the primary implantation as well as to the exchange of the prothesis as the risk of a dislocation of the joint has to be reduced [12].

Post-operative education of the patient can be seen as a means to avoid complications through false behavior.

The most common restrictions can be described as follows using a posterior approach:

– no forced flexion exceeding 90° (for 6 months),
– no forced inner rotation (for 3 months),
– no adduction passing the 0-degree line (for 3 months).

Patients are advised to use a wedge-shaped bolster for the night to avoid a forced adduction during their sleep. There are no restrictions as to the sleeping position although most of the patients cannot lie on the surgical scar as this causes pain.

Crutches should be used until the patient can walk steadily; from then on driving a car should be possible (mostly after 4–6 weeks). A sitting position exceeding 90 degrees is recommended only after the third month after the operation.

Some studies, however, show that the rate of dislocation does not seem to increase without these restrictions [13, 14]. These studies show as well that pre-operative information and education can reduce the risk of a dislocation.

After a TKR (total knee replacement), there are no limitations defined to avoid a dislocation. It is generally only recommended not to put excessive strain on the joint.

There is a great number of programs for the rehabilitation of the patient after arthroplasty. There are, however, great differences in the recommendations for geographical reasons and due to the conviction of the surgeons.

In the majority of the studies [15–19] the number of therapeutic administrations varies from one a day to three a day; that makes it hard to compare.

Furthermore, the progress of rehabilitation depends on the patient's age, his comorbidity and on the surgeon's go-ahead.

Patients who are allowed immediate full weight-bearing show a quicker regeneration and a shorter stay in hospital or in a therapeutic institution [20].

The therapist should always keep in mind the strain an exercise puts on the hip; e.g. the Straight Leg Raise leads to 1.5 up to 1.8 times the bodyweight put on the joint. So this exercise can only be done by patients with full weight-bearing or at least with half its weight [21, 22].

Patients should undergo training at least twice or three times a week. Close supervision and a continuous revision of the training program is strongly recommended.

An individual training program is essential for the success of physiotherapy or occupational therapy as well as massage. A thorough diagnosis is the basis of the steps taken to improve the patient's health.

Manual lymphatic drainage cannot be recommended in a case of septic exchange. Unfortunately, there are no concrete data to be found in the relevant literature.

The main emphasis should be put on the general mobilization, as far as it is advisable, as well as on the mobilization of the scar after the clips or the stitches have been removed, and on the individualized choice of the exercises that are designed to strengthen, mobilize, and stabilize the patient.

The patient's individual living conditions should not be neglected in order to find out what may be done to help him in his daily life, if he or she needs health aids (e.g., a heightened toilet seat, grabs), which activities he or she wants to resume later.

Due to persistent inhibitions and pain most patients have developed mechanisms to avoid such a state before the operation. These mechanisms, however, exert a negative influence on the neighboring joints. That is why it is important to examine and treat these joints, especially the ankle, the knee, the hip, the lumbar vertebrae, and the sacroiliac joint.

Other measures of rehabilitation may help the patient, like group therapies to stabilize the patient's gait, like functional training, as well as physical therapies, e.g., electrotherapy (as long as the local blood circulation is not increased), cryotherapy (in locally defined segments) or heat treatment in the lumbar segment.

It is important to provide the patient with an individually designed program so that he or she can do the exercises at home. But here as well it is difficult to find generally accepted guidelines in the relevant literature.

At present, there are no recommendations for the treatment after septic exchange to be found.

For that reason, a team consisting of medical doctors, of sports scientists and of physiotherapists developed a program—the so-called ENDO Reha—stagemodel after septic knee and hip exchange arthroplasty (developed by Johannes Reich, Nicole Erny, Dr. B. Toussaint and Dr. V. Carrero) (Table 1).

This model comprises five stages that include quadriceps sets, gluteal sets, ankle pumps, and active hip flexion (heel slides) as is the case in most schemes to treat a patient in post-operative rehabilitation [23].

After the operation, most patients remain at the clinic for 14 days (stage 1). The aim at this stage is enable the patient to do transfers independently; increase the range of movement; activate and strengthen muscles; go up and down stairs.

If the patient qualifies and if the healing of the joint has sufficiently progressed, the patient moves on to stage 2.

At the end of the hospital stay, it is recommendable to evaluate the patient's level of independence using the modified IOWA Level of Assistance Scale (mILOAS). On the basis of these data, the functional status of the patient and the status of his or her independence can be assessed, and further measures can be recommended (Tables 1 and 2).

In a survey of 26 functional tests, Terwee et al. [24] found that the ILOAS is the most reliable and most suitable test after arthroplasty. The authors, however, state that more robust data are needed.

The only difference between the two variants lies in the fact that the mILOAS does not measure walking speed but distance, which considerably facilitates the therapist's work.

Table 1 ENDO Reha—Stagemodel® after septic knee-und hip-exchange arthroplasty

ENDO Reha—Stagemodel® after septic knee—und hip—exchange arthroplasty

Stages	Stage 1	Stage 2	Stage 3	Stage 4	Stage 5
Assessments	Assessments to be passed for stage 2 • Good and safe gait with crutches • Go up and downstairs • Do transfers independently • To dress up independently • Activate quadriceps–Straight leg raise • Evaluate the modified Iowa level of assistance scale (ILOAS)	Assessments to be passed for stage 3 • Safe stand with both feet together—At least. 10 s • Safe semi tandem stand—Haltedauer—at least. 10 s • Full tandem stand—at least. 10 s • 5× sit-to-stand test • 4 m walking test = short physical performance battery test (SPPBT) • Timed—Up and go test Passing criteria: • SPPBT result 10–12/12 points • Timed—Up and go test result: Max. 15 s	Assessments to be passed for stage 4 Cours—Parameters: – 5× sit-to-stand test – 4 m walking test – Timed—Up & go test + – Squat—Quality Additional assessments if the patient got a SPBBT score up to 10/12 points and a good quality in squatting: – Single leg stand—At least. 10 s – Single leg squat—at least. 2 s – Modified Y-balance (to the front and to the side—Anterior/posterior-lateral); compare right and left, Passing criteria: – Timed—Up and go test result: Max. 9–12 s – Single leg stand—At least. 10 s – Single leg squat—quality +2 s. In squat position – Y-balance right and left less than 10–15% difference between left and right	Assessments to be passed for stage 5 Cours—Parameters: – 5× sit-to-stand test – 4 m walking test – Timed—Up & go test. + – Squat jump. – Single leg front hop Passing criteria: – Squat jump—Good quality – Single leg front hop—Good quality and max 10% difference in the width of the hop	Sport specific training

| Physical therapy | • Treatment depends on the individual findings
• Mobilization into stand and walk with crutches
• Gait training
• Steps training
• PEACE & LOVE = protection, elevation, avoid anti-Inflammatories, compression, Education & Load, optimism, vascularization, exercise
• Education (Kontraindikationen)
• Learn the activity daily living activities
• Learn how to use the aids for putting socks on, grab things from the ground etc. | • Treatment depends on the individual findings
• Mobilization of the operated joint end of range (consider the precautions for a total hip arthroplasty)
• Scar mobilization
• If necessary treat the higher tension oft he muscles
• Elektrotherapy (for example: TENS quadriceps)
• No manual lymphdrainage,
• Gait training
• Pelvis stabilisation | • Treatment depends on the individual findings
• Continue treatments from stage 2
• ADL training: Getting into the car, transfer from stand—Knee stand—tot he ground, pick up something from the ground without aids, getting into the tub | • Treatment depends on the individual findings
• In this stage training is the most important aim,
• If nessassary continue treatment from stage 1–3 | • In this stage training is the most important aim
• If nessassary continue treatment from stage 1–4
• If the doctor clear to do sport again sport specific training |

Assessments

4 m walking test: < 4.82 s—very good—4 points 4.82–6.20 s—good—3 points 6.21–8.70 s—bad—2 points > 8.70 s—high risk to fall—1 point Distanz not possible—0 points	Balance testing: Normal stands: 10 s. (1 point)—<10 s. (0 point) Semi tandem: 10 s. (1 point)—<10 s. (0 point) Tandem: 10 s. (2 point)—3–9 s. (1 point)— < 3 s. (0 point)
	Timed Up and Go Test (Bohannon et al. 2006): 60–69 years: 9.0 s. 70–79 years: 10.2 s 80–99 years: 12.7 s. (men −5%, women +5%)

(continued)

Table 1 (continued)

5 times sit to stand test:	Single leg stand:	Modified Iowa level of assistance scale:
<11.19 s.—Very good—4 points 11.2–13.69—good—3 points 13.7–16.69—medium—2 points > 16.7—bad—1 point > 60 s. Or test not possible—0 points	2 s.—Passed <2 s.—Not passed	Tests: • Transfer from lying on the back to sit on the bed • Transfer from the bed from sit to stand • 4 m walking test • Go up—and downstairs • Maximum walking distance • Assistive device

Developed by Johannes Reich, Nicole Erny, Dr. B. Toussaint, Dr. V. Carrero

Table 2 Modified Iowa Level of assistance scale

Score	Amount of assistance	Item 1–4	Item 5	Item 6
0	Independent	No assistance is necessary to safety perform the activity (with or without device/aid)	>40 m	No assistive device
1	Standby	Nearby supervision is required; no contact is necessary	26–40 m	1 stick or crutch
2	Minimal	One point of contact is necessary, including helping with the application of the assistive device, getting legs on/off leg rest, and stabilizing the assistive device	10–25 m	2 sticks
3	Morderate	Two points of contact needed (1–2 people)	5–9 m	2 elbow cruthes
4	Maximal	Significant support—3 or more points of contact (>1 person)	3–4 m	2 axillary crutches
5	Failed	Attempted activity but failed with maximal assistance	2 m	Frame (standard or wheelie)
6	Not tested	Test was not attempted due to medical reasons or reasons of safety	<2 m	Gutter/plattform frame, standing lifter, hoist, or unsafe to use aid

Modified Iowa Level of Assistance Scale items: 1-supine to sitting on the edge of the bed, 2-Sit to stand, 3-Walking, 4-Negotiation of one step, 5-Walking distance, 6-Assistive device used. Adapted from Phys Ther. 1995;75(3):169–176, with permission of the American Physical Therapy Association

Literature:
Richard K Shields, Lori J Enloe, Richard E Evans, Kent B Smith, Susan D Steckel; 1995: Reliability, Validity, and Responsiveness of Functional Tests in Patients With Total Joint Replacement. *Physical Therapy*, Volume 75, Issue 3, 1 March 1995, Pages 169–176
Lara A. Kimmel, Jane E. Elliott, James M. Sayer, Anne E. Holland; 1995: Physical Therapy Volume 96, Number 2: Assessing the Reliability and Validity of a Physical Therapy Functional Measurement Tool—the Modified Iowa Level of Assistance Scale—in Acute Hospital Inpatients
Bohannon: A descriptive meta-analyses. Journal of geriatric physical therapy, 2006

In Germany, the medical care at the clinic is often followed by a period of rehabilitation in centers of rehabilitation or as outpatients. The exercises should be done 3–5 days a week, 4–6 hours a session as a requirement of the German health insurance companies.

At stage 2, the emphasis lies on the mobilization in the defined range and on the continued activation and strengthening of the muscles (for relevant exercises and treatment see Tables 1, 3 and 4).

As a further assessment of the patient's status, the patient passes the Short Physical Performance Battery Test (SPPB). This test shows a high validity, reliability, and responsibility in the measurement of the physical function of elderly people [25, 26].

A difference of 0.5 points is classified as a small change, and a difference of 1.0 points as a significant change [26, 27].

Parts of this test battery are

– safe stand with both feet together (position held for 10 s at least),
– safe semi-tandem stand (position held for 10 s at least),

- full tandem stand (position held for 10 s at least),
- five times sit to stand test,
- 4 m walking test.

In addition to this battery, the Timed up and Go Test be assessed (Table 1) The Timed up and Go test is a common test to also evaluate the functional fitness of older patients. The Timed Up and Go (TUG) test was used to measure the time (in seconds) it took the patients to stand up from a chair as quickly and safely as possible, walk 3 m to a line on the floor, and return to the chair. The time is measured from the seated position with a stopwatch. The TUG has been shown to be both reliable and valid [28].

If the patient got a SPPB Test result of minimum 10/12 points and a max. Time of 15 s. in the Timed Up and Go Test the squat needs to be assessed as well. Squatting is a frequent pattern of motion, e.g., when sitting down or standing up, going to the toilet, to bed. For its evaluation and documentation, a marker less tracking software can be used.

The results of these tests and the definition of the stage are also a prediction to choose the best exercises for the patient (Tables 3 and 4).

Table 3 ENDO Reha septic exchange Hip-Arthroplasty—training schedule

	Stage 1	Stage 2	Stage 3	Stage 4	Stage 5
Calf pumps	x				
Heel slides	x	x			
Isometric. M. Glutaei	x	x			
Activation M. Quadriceps	x	x			
Hip mobility exercises—Knee up to 90° in the hip joint	x	x			
Hip abduction/–extension dynamic while standing	x	x			
Gait training with crutches	x	x	x		
Stairs training	x	x	x	x	
Sit to stand	x	x	x	x	
Foot on step and backwards	x	x	x		
Side steps (later with Miniband)	x	x	x	Miniband x x x x	x x x x
Stretch of the hip flexor		x	x	x	
Balance training (Airex pad/Posturomed/single leg stand)		x	x	x	
Single leg stand (later on uneven ground)		x	x	x	
Bridging		x	x	x	
Gait training on treadmill		x	x	x	

Rehabilitation After One-Stage Septic Exchange

Table 3 (continued)

	Stage 1	Stage 2	Stage 3		Stage 4					Stage 5		
Calf raises on step		x	x	x	x	x						
Abduction with a training machine With a short lever arm		x	x	x	x	x	x	x	x	x	x	x
Adduction with a training machine or cable pull with a short lever arm		x	x	x	x	x	x	x	x	x	x	x
Ergometer (at the beginning reduced resistance, short arm, max. 65 R/min.)	10 days	x	X		x	x	x	x	x	x	x	x
Leg press	10 days	x	x		x	x	x	x	x	x	x	x
Hip extension (cable pull over training machine)		x	x	x	x	x	x	x	x	x	x	X
Squat (max 90° hip flexion)		x	x	x	x	x	x	x	x	x	x	x
Leg extension with a training machine		x	x	x	x	x	x	x	x	x	x	x
Star excursion (dorsolateral + lateral)		x	x	x	x	x						
Step up/down			x	x	x	x						
Clamshell			x	x	Mini-band	x	x	x	x	x	x	x
Cross-trainer/ Stairclimber				x	x	x	x	x	x	x	x	x
Bridging (single leg)					x	x	x	x	x	x	x	x
Coordination training (slalom, etc.)						x	x	x	x	x	x	x
Single leg squat (box/ TRX)						x	x	x	x	x	x	x
Lunge						x	x	x	x	x	x	x
Intensive strength training (4 sets à 6–8 reps)										x	x	x

Before the patient start with stage 3, the five times sit to stand test, the 4 m walking test and the Timed Up & Go Test has to be done again as course parameters.

At stage 3, the exercises are intensified, further therapeutic measures taken (see Table 1).

To move to stage 4 you need to passe:

- Timed—Up and Go Test result: max. 9–12 s,
- single leg stand—at least. 10 s,
- single leg squat—quality +2 s. in squat position,
- Y-Balance right and left less than 10–15% difference between left and right.

Table 4 septic exchange ENDO Reha Knee Arthroplasty—training schedule

	Stage 1	Stage 2	Stage 3	Stage 4				Stage 5			
Calf pumps	x	x									
Mobilization with a slider while seated	x	x									
Isometric. M. Glutaei activation	x	x									
Activation of M. Quadriceps	x	x									
Gait training with crutches	x	x	x								
Mobilization in extension/flexion with a pezzi ball supine position	x	x	x								
Balance training (Airex, Posturomed)	X	x	x	x							
Stretching backside (hamstrings)	x	x	x	X							
Steps training	x	x	x	x							
Sit to stand	x	x	x	x							
Calf raises	x	x	x	x	x	x	x	x	x	x	x	x
Side steps (later with Minibands)	x	x	x	Mini-band	x	x	x	x	x	x	x	x
Stepper—Excentric downstairs		X	X	X								
Push into a pezziball		x	x	X								
Hamstring training with a cable pull—Face-down position		x	x	x								
Leg extension with a cable pull/trainings machine		x	x	x								
Single leg stand with uneven ground		x	x	x								
Gait training on a treadmill		x	x	x								
Calf raises		x	x	x	x	x						
Abduction with a trainings machine		x	x	x	x	x	x	x	x	x	x	x
Adduction with a trainings machine		x	x	x	x	x	x	x	x	x	x	x
Ergometer (at the beginning reduced resistance, short arm, max. 65 R/min.)		10 days	x	X	x	x	x	x	x	x	x	x
Leg press		10 days	x	x	x	x	x	x	x	x	x	x
Hip extension training machine		x	x	x	x	x	x	x	x	x	x	X
Squat		x	x	x	x	x	x	x	x	x	x	
Leg curl			x	x	x	x	x	x	x	x	x	

Table 4 (continued)

	Stage 1	Stage 2	Stage 3	Stage 4					Stage 5		
Deadlifts			x	X	X	X	X	X	X	X	X
Lunge			x	X	X	X	X	X	X	X	X
Leg extension			X	x	x	x	x	x	x	x	x
Cross-trainer/Stairclimber			x	x	x	x	x	x	x	x	x
Rowing machine			x	x	X	X	X	X	X	X	X
Single leg squat				x	x	x	x		x	x	x
Intensive strength training [four sets with 6–8 repetitions (reps)]									x	x	x

The patient will be offered further assistance with the exercises in which he failed. And it is necessary to add more extra specific exercises to pass the tests later.

About 12 weeks after the operation, the patient can start training his or her maximum strength (4–5 sets, 6–8 repetitions).

The assessments listed above apply to patients after TKR (total knee replacement) as well as to patients with THR (total hip replacement).

Before moving on to the next stage, there should always be a revision of the goals. A gradual increase of the intensity of the exercises is highly important so as not to impede the healing process of the joint. Tables 3 and 4 show possible exercises to improve the patient's strength and endurance (three times 15–20 repetitions per side and later less repetitions and more sets).

Patients after THR should concentrate on the training of the hip abductors as it is these that stabilize the pelvis when the weight is put on one of the legs; furthermore they guarantee that during the free leg phase the hip avoid the rotational movement. This functions need to be rebuild soon [23, 29]. For the training of these muscles it is advisable to start with isometric exercises. For progression you go on with concentric exercises and the more difficult exercises are the excentric ones (Tables 3 and 4).

As there are no recommendations, programs or schedules for the treatment after septic exchange to be found in the literature (see above), the Helios Endo Rehazentrum Hamburg has developed the Endo Reha—Stage model, complete with a training schedule.

The management plan meets the individual demands of the patients. It takes into account the level of assistance they require. It assesses the patients' ability to perform a number of exercises that are defined by the individual limitations; the further treatment depends on the individual findings.

So the plan undergoes constant revision in accordance with the patient's progress.

References

1. Brown TE, Cui Q, Mihalko WM, et al. Arthritis and arthroplasty: the hip. Philadelphia: Saunders; 2009.
2. Brander VA, Stulberg SD, Chang RW. Rehabilitation following hip and knee arthroplasty. Phys Med Rehabil Clin North Am. 1994;5:815–36.

3. Su EP, Perna M, Boettner F, Mayman DJ, Gerlinger T, Barsoum W, Randolph J, Lee G. A prospective, multi-center, randomised trial to evaluate the efficacy of a cryopneumatic device on total knee arthroplasty recovery. J Bone Joint Surg Br. 2012;94(11):153–6.
4. Ivey M, Johnston RV, Uchida T. Cryotherapy for postoperative pain relief following knee arthroplasty. J Arthroplasty. 1994;9(3):285–90.
5. Desteli EE, Imren Y, Aydın N. Effect of both preoperative and postoperative cryoceutical treatment on hemostasis and postoperative pain following total knee arthroplasty. Int J Clin Exp Med. 2015;8(10):19150–5.
6. Holmström A, Härdin BC. Cryo/Cuff compared to epidural anesthesia after knee unicompartmental arthroplasty: a prospective, randomized, and controlled study of 60 patients with a 6-week follow-up. J Arthroplast. 2005;20(3):316–21.
7. Adie S, Naylor JM, Harris IA. Cryotherapy after total knee arthroplasty: a systematic review and meta-analysis of randomized controlled trials. J Arthroplast. 2010;25(5):709–15.
8. Thienpont E. Does advanced cryotherapy reduce pain and narcotic consumption after knee arthroplasty? Clin Orthop Relat Res. 2014;472(11):3417–23.
9. Okoro T, et al. The use of cryotherapy in the early postoperative perizod after total hip arthroplasty. Ortop Traumatol Rehabil. 2019;21(5):339–48.
10. Iwakiri K, et al. Efficacy of continuous local cryotherapy following total hip arthroplasty. SICOT J. 2019;5:13.
11. Ni S-H, et al. Cryotherapy on postoperative rehabilitation of joint arthroplasty. Knee Surg Sports Traumatol Arthrosc. 2015;23(11):3354–61.
12. Masonis JL, Bourne RB. Surgical approach, abductor function, and total hip arthroplasty dislocation—hip Society and American Association of Hip and Knee Surgeons. Clin Orthop Relat Res. 2002;NO 405:46–53.
13. Peak EL, Parvizi J, Ciminiello M, et al. The role of patient restrictions in reducing the prevalence of early dislocation following total hip arthroplasty. A randomized, prospective study. J Bone Joint Surg Am. 2005;87:247–53.
14. Talbot NJ, Brown JH. N.J Treble: early dislocation after total hip arthroplasty: are postoperative restrictions necessary? J Arthroplasty. 2002;17:1006–8.
15. Henrichs S, Zech A, Schmitt B, Pfeifer K. Die Dosierung der Bewegungstherapie in der Rehabilitation nach Knie- oder Hüft-TEP. Bewegungstherapie GE. 2013;29:11–5.
16. Burton DS, Lmrie SH. Total hip arthroplasty and postoperative rehabilitation. Phys Ther. 1973;53f2:132–40.
17. Chandler HP. Postoperative management and follow-up evaluation. In: Hungerford DS, Krackow K, Kenna R, editors. Total knee arthroplasty-a comprehensive approach. Baltimore: Williams & Wilkins; 1984. p. 1 10–24.
18. Kaye G. The cementless total hip arthroplasty. Physiotherapy. 1982;68(1 2):394–8.
19. Mangine RE. Physical therapy of the knee. New York, NY: Churchill Livingstone; 1988. p. 210–20.
20. Kishida Y, Sugano N, Sakai T, et al. Full weight bearing after cementless total hip arthroplasty. Int Orthop. 2001;25:25–8.
21. Giangarra C, Manske R. Clinical orthopaedic rehabliitation. Amsterdam: Elsevier; 2017. p. 436.
22. Davy DT, Kotzar GM, Brown RH, et al. Telemetric force measurements across the hip and after total arthroplasty. J Bone Joint Surg. 1988;70A:45–50.
23. Enloe LJ, Shields RK, Smith K, et al. Total hip and knee replacement treatment programs: a report using consensus. J Orthop Sports Phys Ther. 1996;23(3–11):8749744.
24. Terwee CB, Mokkink LB, Steultjens MP, et al. Performance based methods for measuring the ohysical function of patients with osteoarthritis of the hip or knee: a systematic review of measurment properties. Rheumatology (Oxford). 2006;45(7):890–902.
25. Freiberger E, de Vreede P, Schoene D, Rydwik E, Mueller VR, Frändin KM, Hopman-Rock M. Performance-based physical function in older community-dwelling persons: a systematic review of instruments. Age Ageing. 2012;41(6):712–21.

26. Treacya D, Hassetta L. The short physical performance battery. Sydney: The George Institute for Global Health, Sydney Medical School, The University of Sydney b Physiotherapy Department, Prince of Wales Hospital, South Eastern Sydney Local Health District c Faculty of Health Sciences The University of Sydney; 2018.
27. Perera S, Mody SH, Woodman RC, Studenski SA. Meaningful change and responsiveness in common physical performance measures in older adults. J Am Geriatr Soc. 2006;54:743–9.
28. Yeung SM, Wessel J, Stratford P, Macdermid J. The timed up and go test for use on an inpatient orthopaedic rehabilitation ward. J Orthop Sports Phys Ther. 2008;38:401–7.
29. Soderberg GL. Kinesiology: applications to pathological motion. Baltimore: Williams & Wilkins; 1986.

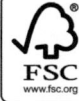

MIX
Papier aus verantwortungsvollen Quellen
Paper from responsible sources
FSC® C105338

If you have any concerns about our products,
you can contact us on
ProductSafety@springernature.com

In case Publisher is established outside the EU,
the EU authorized representative is:
**Springer Nature Customer Service Center GmbH
Europaplatz 3, 69115 Heidelberg, Germany**

Printed by Libri Plureos GmbH
in Hamburg, Germany